STUDY SKILLS
FOR NURSES

Student Survival Skills Series

Survive your nursing course with these essential guides for all student nurses:

Calculation Skills for Nurses
Claire Boyd
9781118448892

Medicine Management Skills for Nurses
Claire Boyd
9781118448854

Clinical Skills for Nurses
Claire Boyd
9781118448779

Care Skills for Nurses
Claire Boyd
9781118657386

Communication Skills for Nurses
Claire Boyd and Janet Dare
9781118767528

Study Skills for Nurses
Claire Boyd
9781118657430

STUDY SKILLS
FOR NURSES

Claire Boyd
RGN, Cert Ed
Practice Development Trainer

with contributions by
Beverley Murray
MCLIP, Level 3 NVQ in Direct Training
and Support
E-resources and Training Manager

WILEY Blackwell

This edition first published 2014
© 2014 by John Wiley & Sons, Ltd

Registered office:
John Wiley & Sons, Ltd, The Atrium, Southern Gate, Chichester, West Sussex, PO19 8SQ, UK

Editorial offices:
9600 Garsington Road, Oxford, OX4 2DQ, UK
The Atrium, Southern Gate, Chichester, West Sussex, PO19 8SQ, UK
111 River Street, Hoboken, NJ 07030-5774, USA

For details of our global editorial offices, for customer services and for information about how to apply for permission to reuse the copyright material in this book please see our website at www.wiley.com/wiley-blackwell

Library of Congress Cataloging-in-Publication Data
Boyd, Claire, author.
  Study skills for nurses / Claire Boyd ; with contributions by Beverley Murray.
    1 online resource. – (Student survival skills)
  Includes bibliographical references and index.
  Summary: "A concise, pocket-sized companion on study skills, aimed at student nurses beginning their course, looking for a refresher on key skills, or returning to further study"–Provided by publisher.
  Description based on print version record and CIP data provided by publisher; resource not viewed.
  ISBN 978-1-118-65740-9 (Adobe PDF) – ISBN 978-1-118-65741-6 (ePub) – ISBN 978-1-118-65743-0 (paper)
  I. Murray, Beverley, contributor. II. Title.
  [DNLM: 1. Education, Nursing–methods–Handbooks. 2. Test Taking Skills–methods–Handbooks. WY 49]
  RT71
  610.73–dc23
                                                                                          2014023323

A catalogue record for this book is available from the British Library.

Wiley also publishes its books in a variety of electronic formats. Some content that appears in print may not be available in electronic books.

Cover image courtesy of Visual Philosophy
Chapter opener image: © iStockphoto.com/pilip7
Cover design by Visual Philosophy

Set in 9/12pt Trade Gothic LT Std by Aptara Inc., New Delhi, India
Printed and bound in Malaysia by Vivar Printing Sdn Bhd

1 2014

Contents

CONTENTS

Preface

This book is designed to assist the student healthcare worker in the 'how to' of study skills, while incorporating healthcare-related information to further assist the learner in their course.

It is designed to give a quick, snappy overview of study skills techniques and strategies. Students enter academic study from a variety of starting points, such as straight from college/school. In this case they may already have many skills to equip them in the world of advanced study. However, some students may enter their nurse training after many years away from academic study. This book, with its links to the nurse training programme, will offer something for all, be it initial study skills information to assist the new learner or useful information to assist all those entering the health profession.

The book incorporates many exercises to check understanding, and is laid out in a simple to follow step-by-step approach. Chapters end with quizzes to relate everything learned to practice. It has been compiled by quotes and tips from student nurses themselves; it is a book by students for students.

Claire Boyd
Bristol
April 2014

Introduction

Hello, my name is Claire Boyd and I am a Practice Development Trainer, working for one of the largest teaching hospitals in the south west of England, in one of Europe's most modern hospital environments: Southmead Hospital, Bristol.

It took a lot of hard work to achieve my lifelong ambition of becoming a nurse. I have also studied for my Certificate in Education and as a holistic therapist for massage, aromatherapy and other well-being courses. I am not a quick learner, more of a 'plodder', and at university it was important for me to find a means of study that would suit me. It also had to be around my family and my other commitments (I was fostering children at the start of my nurse training; 44 of in all, but not all at the same time)!

On my first day at university, and as the enormity of the next couple of years hit home, I realised that I would have to get myself organised. I purchased a book on study skills which explained that I would need to study during my optimum learning times when I would be 'fresh and alert'. This quickly enabled me to see that 'one fit does not suit all'. When fresh I would be working on the wards and I was unable to find any helpful study skills book that really understood learning from the nursing perspective.

I was able to find my own learning plan, usually from 12 midnight until 2 a.m., which most literature will tell you is 'how not to do it'. This was the only time I could study in a quiet environment, when all the family were in bed, and I could really learn. Some people like to have music or the television on when they are studying, but I need absolute quiet. You take your life in your own hands if you talk to me when I have my nose in an academic book! This taught me the importance of finding your own groove, and what works best for you, the individual.

Keeping to the theme of study skills books on the market, many student nurses tell me that these books mainly do not cater for the student nurse, as they tell me 'we are not the same as other university students'. These are some of the reasons they give.

- When on placement, we are working full time and have to study around those hours.
- Working in our clinical placements we have the added pressure of being responsible for the patients' well-being.
- We are accountable and responsible for our own actions.
- Every day is different; there is so much to learn.
- Nursing is a very demanding job.

(Thanks to Megan Powell, Rosalind Broome and Elizabeth Smart, second year nursing students at the University of the West of England, 2013.)

Studying at university is all about taking responsibility: you are no longer at school or college, where someone is keeping you motivated and nagging you to keep to deadlines. Similarly, studying to become a nurse is like no other university course, as you are expected to work shifts as well as attend lectures, seminars and tutorials. Coupled with this, nurses are required to submit assignments and case studies, have competencies signed off in the workplace, produce reflective pieces and attend 'bedside' teaching sessions! There is also the nursing portfolio in which a student keeps all certificates and other paperwork, ready for attending interviews for nursing jobs, and for the Nursing and Midwifery Council requirements beyond.

Keep with it: nursing is a wonderful, rewarding job, with so many branches in whichever area takes your fancy, such as adult nursing, maternity, paediatric nursing, mental health nursing, learning disabilities, district nursing, working in clinics and GP surgeries, specialising in cardiology, high dependency, orthopaedics, neurosurgery…the list is endless. Table 1 shows what working in ten of these specialities will involve for you, the carer.

Table 1 What nursing work involves

Branch of nursing	What's involved?
Adult nursing	Being part of a busy multidisciplinary team The use of initiative and observation Working in a demanding and fast-changing environment Assessing A willingness to take responsibility for people's well-being Continued learning throughout your career

Branch of nursing	What's involved?
Mental health nursing	Autonomy in planning and delivering care in a healthcare team Opportunities to specialise in areas such as drug or alcohol misuse The ability to empathise with people The use of excellent communication skills Liaising with the patient's family or carers Dealing with occasional aggression in a sensitive and effective way
Children's nursing	The ability to work with those who may be too young to express what's wrong An awareness that a child's health can rapidly take a turn for the worse and manage the situation Using communication skills other than words Working in partnership with the patient's parents, carers and/or siblings Parent, carers and/or sibling education
Learning disability nursing	The use of patience, sensitivity and excellent interpersonal skills The willingness to be adaptable, flexible and act as advocate for those you are supporting The ability to work in a demanding and stressful environment Great satisfaction when someone has learned a new skill
District nursing	Working with a variety of people as part of a team, such as GPs and social services as well as working alone Good organisational skills Helping patients with personal hygiene Carrying out health checks and delivering health promotion programmes Patient education Monitoring health
Neonatal nursing	Being a source of support to the baby's family Taking an active role as part of the multidisciplinary team in looking after the child Empathy The competence to work in a busy, technical environment

(continued)

Table 1 *(Continued)*

Branch of nursing	What's involved?
Health visiting	Working with people who have disabilities or chronic health problems Supporting new mothers in the care and development in their babies Health promotion Good organisational skills The ability to work independently for much of the time Working in occasional challenging situations
Practice nursing	Health screening Family planning Treating small wounds Assisting with minor operations and procedures Running vaccination clinics Managing well-woman clinics Supporting the healthcare team in monitoring health conditions, e.g. diabetes
Prison nursing	Delivering health care in a custodial setting The use of excellent interpersonal skills Developing position and professional relationships with prisoners Dealing with substance abuse and/or mental health problems
School nursing	Carrying out screening programmes Providing health-related information Administering immunisations Providing health and sex education A non-judgemental approach Running health promotion or drop in surgeries
Midwifery	Being a source of support in preparing women for delivery of new life Working in partnership with clients throughout all stages of pregnancy, labour and the early post-natal period The ability to work independently: in the community, clinics, children's centres, GP surgeries Working as part of a multidisciplinary team Good organisation skills Good interpersonal skills Working in occasional challenging situations

Source: adapted from *Careers in Nursing* (www.nhscareers.nhs.uk).

I have been fortunate to have taught many student nurses and it has been with their help that this book, and others in the series (*Calculation Skills, Clinical Skills, Medicine Management Skills, Care Skills* and *Communication Skills*), have been developed; in short, they told me what they wanted included in the books. It is a book for nursing students, and other healthcare professionals wishing to study, such as assistant practitioners, operating department practitioners, healthcare assistants and qualified nurses, giving tips and pointers along the way.

All chapters contain healthcare examples and incorporate student nurses' tips and advice throughout. In short, this book is not a generic study skills book. By being a specifically nurse study skills book – one of its unique properties – the learner benefits not just from acquiring study skills but can also benefit from nurse-related information. For example, while learning about mind mapping techniques in Chapter 6 you will also be introduced to the patient safety concept of implementing 'human factors' in health care. Also, while undertaking the Test your Knowledge section in Chapter 10 you will learn about natural rubber latex allergy. The contents are presented in a style as to make you feel that the tutor is sitting right next to you, helping you along the way.

To assist you with your studies a year planner is included at the end of the book. It is something the student nurses requested to enable them to plan their shift dates around their university lectures, seminars, tutorials and exam and assignment 'due dates', and it can be viewed at a quick glance.

Bibliography

NHS Careers (2012) *Careers in Nursing.* www.nhscareers.nhs.uk.
Nursing and Midwifery Council (2008) *The Code: Standards of Conduct, Performance and Ethics for Nurses and Midwives.* Nursing and Midwifery Council, London; www.nmc-uk.org/code.
Nursing and Midwifery Council (2011) *The PREP Handbook.* NMC, London; www.nmc-uk.org.

Acknowledgements

As always, first acknowledgements go to the student nurses who have helped to make this book possible. As with the other books in the Student Survival Skills Series, it is their tips and quotes that have been used throughout the book.

Acknowledgements also go to Beverley Murray (E-resources and Training Manager) for her contribution in Chapter 4 and the critical reading section in Chapter 5, and to Lesley Greig (Library Service Manager). Thanks also to Kim Hacker (Skills for Life Facilitator) at North Bristol NHS Trust for her help and guidance. Also to Jane Hadfield (Head of Learning and Development) and to all my friends and colleagues in the Staff Development Department at North Bristol NHS Trust.

Thanks to NHS Employers for the use of The New NHS in 2013: What it Means for You infographic in Appendix 4.

Thanks also go to Magenta Styles (Executive Editor at Wiley Blackwell) for first approaching me about this exciting project, Madeleine Hurd (Associate Commissioning Editor), Catriona Cooper and James Schultz (Project Editors), Nik Prowse (freelance copy-editor) for copy-editing the manuscript, Mirjana Misina (Project Manager) and to Simon Boyd for indexing all my books for me.

This book is dedicated to my family: my lovely husband Rob, and Simon, Louise and David. Thank you for supporting me in my book-writing foray and for all your help and assistance.

Chapter 1

LEARNING AT UNIVERSITY

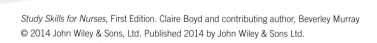

Study Skills for Nurses, First Edition. Claire Boyd and contributing author, Beverley Murray
© 2014 John Wiley & Sons, Ltd. Published 2014 by John Wiley & Sons Ltd.

LEARNING OUTCOMES

By the end of this chapter you will have an understanding of university learning, your university course, some key terms and the learning process.

First of all, congratulations on achieving your place at university to begin your nurse training (or other healthcare-associated course). Some of you will have entered university straight from school or college, others may be coming back to academic study after many years. Your initial concerns about the course will vary depending on your particular circumstances. For instance, for some new students first thoughts will be about finances, accommodation, child care, balancing study with family life and other responsibilities. Some of you will wonder how you'll manage when confronted with blood and gore, death and dying. And let's be honest, some of you will be more concerned initially about the social side to university, and about the possibilities of making lifelong friends. This diversity is one of the rich and fulfilling elements of university education, and where we can all learn from each others' experiences, skills and strengths.

Whoever you are or whatever your age, this book will assist you in making better use of your study time. Study skills evolve and mature through practice and as you move through your course.

KEY DIFFERENCES BETWEEN SCHOOL/COLLEGE AND UNIVERSITY EDUCATION

If you have come into university education straight from school or college, you will notice that there is much more autonomy: no one will be nagging you to get assignments in on time or competences signed off. The emphasis is on you, the individual, and on self-responsibility and self-management. You will need to organise your study time around your clinical placements and prioritise different tasks (such as competency assessments, reflection and assignments).

One of the most important aspects of university study is the work you undertake independently of the tutors, either on your own or with other students. Sometimes you may be assessed on the outcomes of your group projects.

Another difference with university education is that teachers are usually referred to as tutors. Tutors will help you develop and provide support, and in addition you will have mentors, or preceptors, in your clinical placements to help guide you through your nurse education.

THE LEARNING PROCESS

To learn effectively you need to be aware of the four main factors of the learning process. This awareness will improve how you learn:

- **wanting to learn:** you will need a sense of purpose and motivation;
- **learning by doing:** you will need to practice (i.e. making hospital beds), perhaps making mistakes at first;
- **receiving feedback:** you will learn from both positive and negative feedback;
- **reflection:** you will also learn from reviewing and evaluating what has been learned, and drawing conclusions.

DEVELOPING YOUR LEARNING SKILLS

To get the best out of your university course you will need to develop and enhance a wide range of key skills, such as:

- time management,
- prioritising,
- team work and working with others,
- oral presentations,

- note-taking,
- communicating through written essays/assignments and reports,
- understanding numbers and charts,
- problem solving,
- reading effectively and efficiently,
- revision and exam skills,
- using assessment: self-assessment and peer assessment, and using feedback,
- information technology,
- using the library and gathering information.

These core skills will not only assist you during your course, but also when you are seeking employment. These are the **transferable skills** that you will use throughout your nursing career.

KEY TERMS FOR UNIVERSITY

At university you may encounter some terms or phrases that you haven't heard before. See Activity 1.1: how many or these do you know already?

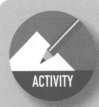

Activity 1.1

ACTIVITY

Do you understand these key terms?

Lecture
Seminar
Tutorial
Practicals
Self-guided study
Computer-aided learning
Assessment

YOUR NURSING COURSE

Once you are on a nurse training programme, you will divide your time between university and supervised placements in local hospitals and the social care setting (the community). Most courses are full time and take 3 years to complete. Many universities offer part-time pre-registration nursing courses, which usually last for 5 or 6 years. As your course progresses you will be expected to deliver practical care, such as:

- checking and recording temperatures,
- measuring blood pressure and respiratory rates,
- helping doctors with physical examinations,
- giving medications and injections,
- collecting blood for transfusion,
- cleaning and dressing wounds,
- using hi-tech medical equipment.

These skills initially can only be performed under supervision with a qualified member of staff. You can conduct them on your own when you have had the competencies signed off and been deemed competent.

As a nurse, you will usually work 37.5 hours per week, which will include evenings, weekends, night shifts and bank holidays. Care does not stop for the patient over these times, so nor do your working hours.

In September 2011 pre-registration nurse education was moved from diploma to degree programmes. Since September 2013 students have only been able to qualify as a nurse by studying at degree level.

During your first year at university you will follow the common foundation programme, which includes an introduction to the four branches of nursing (adult nursing, paediatric nursing, mental health nursing, learning disabilities nursing) and maternity care. You will further be introduced to observational, communication and caring skills, study anatomy, physiology, psychology, sociology and social policy, and learn core practical caring skills. Over the remaining 2 years you will specialise in your chosen branch of nursing and work in the relevant clinical placement areas.

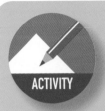

Activity 1.2

The NHS Careers website (www.nhscareers.nhs.uk) states that to pursue a successful career in nursing you need to possess five key skills: what do you think they are?

Nurses also need to possess certain values and behaviours. These are part of the culture of compassionate care and are called the six Cs: care, compassion, competence, communication, courage and commitment (Department of Health and NHS Commissioning Board 2012).

TAKING RESPONSIBILITY

You may feel that your computer skills are not up to speed, but do not ignore this problem. They are essential education skills in the modern world. Universities expect assignments to be word processed; handwritten assignments are a thing of the past. It is important for you to have an understanding of commonly used technological terms. See how many of the terms listed in Activity 1.3 that you know.

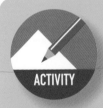

Activity 1.3

It is important for you to have an understanding of information and computing technology (or ICT). What do these terms mean?

application	modem
attachment	operating system
broadband	output devices
browser	portable document format (PDF)
compact disc (CD)	processor
download	program
DVD	RAM memory
file	router
firewall	software
folder	spam
forum	uniform resource locator (URL)
gigabyte (GB)	universal serial bus (USB)
hard disc	USB flash drive
input device	virus
internet	web
Internet Explorer	web browser
ISP (internet service provider)	wireless fidelity (WiFi)
megabyte (MB)	window
memory	Windows

During your course you will have ICT training. Embracing this skill will enable you to gather information at your fingertips using the worldwide web (from reputable sources only, of course). Chapter 4 goes into detail on how to conduct effective internet searches.

PRACTICAL ARRANGEMENTS

At the start of your university course it is important to establish a place to study, where you can work undisturbed. The area should have plenty of space for you to spread your books and papers, where you have access to study aids and resources. It should have a good light source and not be too hot or cold. Now let's be realistic, most of us don't have these facilities, so we must make do with what we have. You will also require access to a computer, either at home or in the university. It is important to mention here that as well as support from fellow students on your course, you will also need the support of those closest to you. Let me paint you a picture:

> Student: OMG! Just had my draft assignment back and I have so much work to do by Monday's submission date! Why did I leave it all so late?
>
> Significant other: What! The weather's meant to be lovely this weekend, so I thought we could go to the beach. You haven't had a weekend off in ages!
>
> Student: You've got to be joking! I'll need to spend the weekend completing my work!
>
> Significant other: Surely a few tweaks won't take all weekend!
>
> Student: I've got a lot more to do than just a few tweaks!
>
> Significant other: (through gritted teeth) Never mind.
>
> Student: (ironically) Thanks for your support.

This is where you have to decide on your priorities: your choice could affect your marks and your chosen career.

STUDENTS WITH DYSLEXIA

Some students have to contend with a learning difficulty while studying in higher education. This learning difficulty could be related to maths and numbers – known as dyscalculus – or relate to words, which is called dyslexia. Table 1.1 gives an overview of dyslexia.

It is important to inform your tutor of any learning difficulties that you have, and to inform your mentor while on clinical placement. This way you can gain the correct support through Student Services.

Table 1.1 Dyslexia: range of difficulties

Area	Problems
Speech and language	Numeracy (language of maths) Phonological skills (rhyming sounds, sounds and blends) Reading (tracking) Spelling, remembering words, sequencing, syllables, using wrong words Sequencing (letters in words and words in sentences)
Memory	Poor short-term memory Trouble with following instructions, spelling patterns, names
Motor skills	Clumsy, poor pencil control Poor organisational skills (lateness, untidy, disorganised)
Emotional and behaviour	Low self esteem (risk of failure, low confidence) Can be aggressive, disruptive or confrontational

Case Study 1.1

Not long ago I was facilitating the calculations test at my trust. This is taken by student nurses to prove their maths competence so that they can attend the Intravenous (IV) Study Day. Only then can a nurse be signed off for the ability to administer IV drugs (after competency assessments have been achieved). Students are asked to tell me in advance if they have any learning difficulties. Individuals who do may request tests on coloured paper or have extra time for tests. At the end of this particular test one newly qualified nurse was referred and I received an email later that day informing me that the nurse was dyslexic and should have received extra time for the test. I went to see her on the ward and took issue with the fact that she had not informed me of her learning needs. She said, 'Yes – I like to keep my learning disability secret, so that no one knows!' A Practice Development Trainer cannot assist students with learning needs if they're kept a secret. The nurse did pass her test after steps were taken to support her.

The moral of this story is to be honest about any learning needs you have. We can only help you if we know about them.

DEADLINES

Universities are not flexible about their deadlines. Your university will have formal mechanisms for arranging extensions if you have exceptional circumstances as to why you are unable to hand in your work on time. You should also discuss this with your tutor. You will be asked to provide evidence of the extenuating circumstances, such as a doctor's certificate. Exceptional circumstances do happen. I needed to have my appendix removed during my own nurse training. To cover the time I spent in hospital having my surgery and recovering afterwards I applied for and received an extension for an assignment.

KEEPING GOING

Much of your university work will require you to work on your own. This does not mean that a group of students can't set up a study support group, exchanging ideas and interpreting assignment questions. But when you do work on your own it may be difficult to keep yourself motivated. One student informed me that they could not get motivated to start work on assignments until the deadline was almost upon them; only then would the adrenaline run and they start to work! Others have informed me that they start gathering information the moment they get the assignment. At university, you may get given all your assignments and deadlines for a module together, with the same submission date. Then you need to prioritise your workload.

GATHERING AND SHARING INFORMATION

Using social media is perhaps the most common way in which you will share information with your fellow students. College lecturers and professors also use social media to communicate with students via podcasts, video, wikis and blogs for their classes.

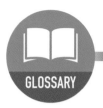

Podcast

Audio content on a website that can be transferred onto an audio player, such as an iPod or other MP3 player.

Wiki

Information website that allows individuals to add, modify or delete web page content.

Blog

Discussion or informational site published on the world wide web.

The social media sites most widely used by students, to name just a few, are Facebook, Twitter and YouTube. They can also be accessed via devices such as laptops, iPads, smartphones and other tablets. New media tools are constantly being developed to help students network, communicate and share information and knowledge with their peers. Social media may also be used by the university itself to showcase students' work as well as to promote events and pass on information to students.

USEFUL WEBSITES FOR NURSES

Universities will usually provide you with useful websites during your training to support you through your course. There are many computer software programs to assist students in their studies, such as referencing packages whereby you may just type in an author's name and initials and the correct referencing system is produced for you. Universities often also develop their own useful resources on referencing using the Harvard system for different types of source, such as books, journals, electronic media (e.g. television broadcasts), electronic sources (e.g. websites), publications by government and official bodies (e.g. Nursing and Midwifery Council, Department of Health) and others (e.g. newspapers) and you should take full advantage of this.

Table 1.2 gives some useful websites for nurses, from around the world.

Table 1.2 Useful nursing websites

Website	URL	Information
NurseZone	www.nursezone.com	Features, journals and information
Nurse.com	www.nurse.com	For adult nurses, midwives, community and all sectors of nursing
Forensic Nurse	www.theforensicnurse.com	Articles and news
PubMed	www.ncbi.nlm.nih.gov/pubmed	US government database for medical and health science resources
Medscape Nurses	www.medscape.com/nurses	News and resources
Nursing Times	www.nursingtimes.net	News, features and jobs
World Wide Wounds	www.worldwidewounds.com	Discusses dressings/materials, etc.
Allnurses	http://allnurses.com	Site for camaraderie and guidance
Nursing Link	http://nursinglink.monster.com	Nursing community that offers forums and education links
NurseConnect	www.nurseconnect.com	Network for career advancement
NurseGroups	www.nursegroups.com	Camaraderie in your nursing field
Forum for Nurses	www.nursingforum.co.uk	Learn about the different specialties in nursing
Nurses Reconnect	www.nursesreconnected.com	To liaise with your friends and peers in health care
Nursespage	https://twitter.com/thenursespage	Discussion site with blogs, etc.
Everyday Nurses	www.everydaynurses.com	Convene with your colleagues
NurseChat	www.facebook.com/pages/NURSE-CHAT	Talk about jobs, education and lots more

Website	URL	Information
AORN	www.aorn.org	Association of Perioperative Registered Nurses
Association of Rehabilitation Nurses	www.rehabnurse.org	Association of Rehabilitation Nurses
International Council of Nurses	www.icn.ch	Organisation promoting the profession of nursing and nurses
National Black Nurses Association	www.nbna.org	Organisation to promote black nurses
Cancer Nursing	www.cancernursing.org	For free courses, news and forum discussions
Medi-Smart	www.medi-smart.com	Site for nursing education resources
The Foundation Center for Nursing Research	www.ninr.nih.gov	US site for those wishing to pursue nursing research
SkillStat Learning	www.skillstat.com	Site full of learning tools
RN.com	www.rn.com	Continuing education and resources
ERNursey	www.ernursey.blogspot.com	Blog site for those in emergency nursing
Clinical Cases and Images	clinicalcases.org	Articles and interesting information
Nightingale Letters	www.bl.uk/onlinegallery/onlineex/histtexts/flonight/index.html	Interesting information from Nightingale's letters
Care Plans	www.nhs.uk/Planners/Yourhealth/Pages/Careplan.aspx	Discussions about care planning
Nursing Ethics	www.nmc-uk.org/Publications/Standards/The-code/Introduction	Learn about codes of ethics and other useful information
Nursing Calculators	www.manuelsweb.com/nursing.htm	Calculators helping with working out drug dosages

(continued)

Table 1.2 *(Continued)*

Website	URL	Information
Clinical Calculators	www.mims.co.uk/Calculators/	Includes pregnancy due-date calculator and measurement converter
Nursing Theory	www.coxhealth.com/nursingtheoryandtheorists	Contains many nursing links
Medical Practice Guidelines	http://med.oxfordradcliffe.net/guidelines	Information on many medical conditions
Facts and Comparisons	www.factsandcomparisons.com	Looks at drugs and drug information
NursingFun	www.nursingfun.com	Jokes, games and nursing-related fun
School Nurse News	www.schoolnursenews.org	A good site for keeping abreast of all the news in this field of nursing

C-R-E-A-M STRATEGY

Cream is not just for cats! (Figure 1.1) Cottrell (1999) recommends the C-R-E-A-M strategy as a means of developing your study skills (Table 1.3).

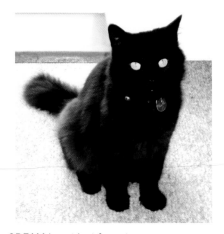

Figure 1.1 CREAM is not just for cats

Table 1.3 C-R-E-A-M strategy

C = Creative	Have the confidence to use your individual strategies and styles and apply imagination to your learning
R = Reflective	Be able to sit with your experience, analyse and evaluate your own performance and draw lessons from it
E = Effective	Organise your space, time, priorities, state of mind and resources to the maximum benefit
A = Active	Be personally involved and doing things, physically and mentally, to help to make sense of what you learn
M = Motivated	Be aware of your own desired outcomes; keep yourself on track using short and long-term goals

Source: Cottrell (1999).

KEY POINTS

- Key differences between schools/colleges and university education
- The learning process
- Developing your learning skills
- Key terms for university
- Your nursing course
- Taking responsibility
- Practical arrangements
- Learning difficulties
- Deadlines
- Keeping going
- Social media and websites
- C-R-E-A-M strategy

TEST YOUR KNOWLEDGE

Here is a gentle activity for you.

Write your important dates on your yearly planner (at the back of this book). Write in shift dates (when they begin), assignment-submission dates, university dates, dates when you are giving presentations and one-to-one meeting with your tutor. Start to utilise this organisation tool.

Bibliography

Cottrell, S. (1999) *The Study Skills Handbook*. MacMillan, Basingstoke.

Department of Health and NHS Commissioning Board (2012) *Developing the Culture of Compassionate Care: Creating a New Vision for Nurses, Midwives and Care-givers*. Consultation/discussion paper. Department of Health, London.

Open University (2011) *Using a Computer to Support Your Study*. Open University, Milton Keynes.

Selwyn, N. (2007) The use of computer technology in university teaching and learning: a critical perspective. *Journal of Computer Assisted Learning* 23, 83–94.

Websites

National Leadership and Innovation Agency for Healthcare, www.nliah.wales.nhs.uk

Nursing and Midwifery Council (NMC), www.nmc-uk.org

Skills for Health, www.skillsfor health.org.uk

Chapter 2

. . . .

UNDERSTANDING HOW YOU LEARN

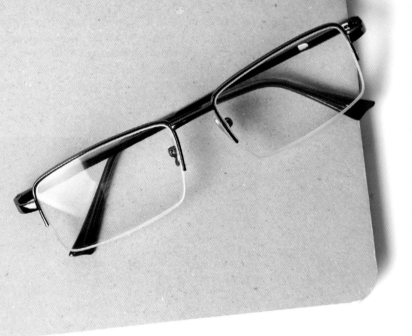

Study Skills for Nurses, First Edition. Claire Boyd and contributing author, Beverley Murray
© 2014 John Wiley & Sons, Ltd. Published 2014 by John Wiley & Sons Ltd.

LEARNING OUTCOMES

By the end of this chapter you will have an understanding of your own preferred learning style and the VARK system of perception, and how to use these beneficially to suit your own learning needs.

In Chapter 1 you learned that studying at university is very different from studying at school or college. It's important to have fun while at university, as long as you keep focused: work before play! (See Figure 2.1.)

Of course, it is important to have developed a reliable study ethos – which will stand you in good stead during your course – if you have come into nursing straight from school or college. We all study in different ways: some of us work at a steady, systematic way, whereas others may prefer to study during long or short intensive bursts. Some of us read text and look for the underlying meaning, known as **deep learning**. This is often required for studying at university level. Others may read a text and try to remember its contents, known as **surface learning**. Some of us are quite happy to read words, but may struggle to read tables, numbers and graphs.

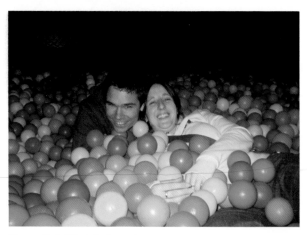

Figure 2.1 Work before play

To get the best out of your study it is useful to know your **preferred learning style**. You may be thinking, what does this mean? Don't worry, all will be revealed a little later on! In the meanwhile, just for a bit of fun, have a go at Activity 2.1.

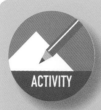

Activity 2.1 Preferred learning style

Memorise the line below. Then, 1 hour later, without looking, see if you can recite the numbers and letters in their correct order.

1991200153mep

Source: www.esrcsocietytoday.ac.uk (Economic and Social Research Council 2013).

Have a look at Activity 2.1 again. Now that the line in the activity makes sense, it becomes easier to remember. In other words, the better you understand something, the easier it is to learn. Now try Activity 2.2.

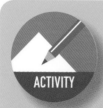

Activity 2.2

Try to spot the pattern in this group of letters:

aobocodoeofpgphpipjp

How did you do? The better you are at identifying and remembering patterns in what you are studying, the better and more successful you could be in your studies. You may be wondering what on earth Activities 2.1 and 2.2 have to do with study skills. Well, if you are ever asked to *compare and contrast* two articles or reports, it is important that you can pull out the similarities and key themes, and the differences between them. In other words, to find the pattern.

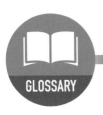

Compare

To look for the differences and similarities between two written documents.

Contrast

To find only the differences and to present the results in an orderly fashion.

Lastly, have a go at looking at the pattern in Activity 2.3.

Activity 2.3

Can you establish a pattern in the pictures?

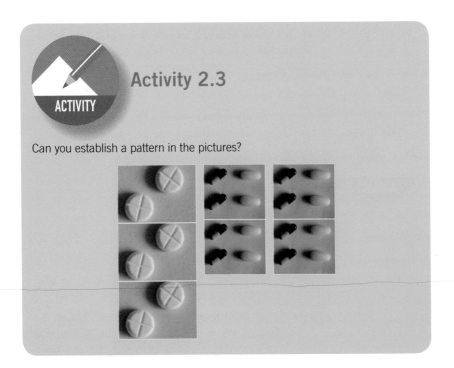

This was a simple pattern, but the aim was to establish whether you found the visual activity easier than the ones with words. We all have our own preferred way of taking in information: our **learning preferences**. Once you know your own learning style, you can adapt your learning to meet your needs.

YOUR LEARNING STYLE

There has been much written about learning styles and many competing theories, but one of the most well known was developed by Honey and Mumford (1992). There are sites on the internet that allow you to establish your own learning style. Learners answer a set of questions to establish whether their learning style is predominantly as **an activist, a reflector, a theorist or a pragmatist, or a** combination of these. A combination is ideal, as it gives a good balance. The description of each of the learning styles in Table 2.1 will give you an idea of your preferred learning style.

Table 2.1 Your learning style

Learning style	Strengths	Weaknesses
Activists	Flexible and open minded; happy to have a go; happy to be exposed to new situations, Optimistic about anything new and therefore unlikely to resist change.	Tendency to take the immediately obvious action without thinking; often take unnecessary risks; tendency to do too much themselves and hog the limelight; rush into action without sufficient preparation; get bored with implementation/consolidation.
Reflectors	Careful, thorough and methodical, thoughtful, good at listening to others and assimilating information; rarely jump to conclusions.	Tendency to hold back from direct participation; slow to make up their minds and reach a decision; tendency to be too cautious and not take enough risks; not assertive: not particularly forthcoming and have no 'small talk'.

(continued)

Table 2.1 *(Continued)*

Learning style	Strengths	Weaknesses
Theorists	Logical 'vertical' thinkers; rational and objective; good at asking probing questions; disciplined approach.	Restricted in lateral thinking; low tolerance for uncertainty, disorder and ambiguity; intolerant of anything subjective or intuitive; full of 'shoulds, oughts and musts'.
Pragmatists	Keen to test things out in practice; practical; down to earth; realistic; businesslike: get straight to the point; technique orientated.	Tendency to reject anything without an obvious application; not very interested in theory or basic principles; tendency to seize on the first expedient solution to a problem; impatient with waffle; on balance, task orientated.

Adapted from Honey and Mumford (1992).

But what does all this mean and how can we use this information to our advantage? Well, it's all about dovetailing each learning activity with the individual's preferred learning style. That's why learning institutions use a variety of teaching methods: to accommodate the different learning styles.

HOW TO IMPROVE YOUR PREFERRED LEARNING STYLE

- **Activist-style learners:** Practise initiating conversations with your new peers and patients when in clinical placement.
- **Pragmatist-style learners:** Study learning techniques that others use. When you discover something they do well, emulate them.
- **Theorist-style learners:** Practise spotting inconsistencies/ weaknesses in other people's arguments. Go through reports highlighting inconsistencies.
- **Reflector-style learners:** Practise drawing up lists for and against a particular course of action. Take a contentious issue and produce balanced arguments from both points of view.

PERCEIVING INFORMATION

From the moment we wake in the morning, we start to gather information about the world around us. Even when we study, we utilise all our senses. The VARK system, devised by Fleming (2006) helps us to understand our strengths and weaknesses in regard to perception (Box 2.1).

Box 2.1 The VARK system

Visual (sight)
Auditory (hearing)
Reading
Kinaesthetic (using movement and touch)

Visual learners may learn best by seeing, Auditory learners may absorb more information that they hear or have discussed, some individuals may learn more by reading a book, whereas kinaesthetic learners may learn more during practical classes with hands-on- activities. I am very much a visual learner.

As in all areas of life, we should strive to make the most of our strengths and build on our weaker areas. Knowing how we perceive the information we are gathering during our study is all very well, but we need to put this information into practice and make it work to our advantage.

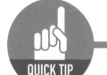

QUICK TIP

Visual learners should try the following.

1 **Choose visual materials, such as books with pictures, charts and maps.**
2 **Use a highlighter pen to highlight your notes.**
3 **Use coloured stick tabs to mark text books.**
4 **Use spider maps, illustrations and models to aid your learning.**

(continued)

5   Study in quiet places away from noise and visual disturbances.
6   Visualise information as a picture, where able.
7   Skim-read to get an overview before reading in detail.

Auditory learners should try the following.

1   Use a tape recorder or digital voice recorder, if possible, instead of making notes.
2   Discuss your ideas verbally.
3   Participate in discussions and debates.
4   Make speeches and presentations.
5   Create mnemonics to aid memory.
6   Record yourself speaking and listen to your ideas played back.

Kinaesthetic learners should try the following.

1   Move around to learn new things.
2   Stand up to work.
3   Skim-read before reading in detail.
4   Take frequent study breaks and time-outs.

Whatever your natural learning preference, there will be times when you need to adapt this preference, moving outside of your comfort zone. Learning preferences are useful to know, helping you to become more effective in your studies, but they can be adapted to suit the task. In other words, you can improve your effectiveness by balancing your approach to your learning and therefore making the most of your learning potential. If you are a visual learner, preferring to watch, there may be times when you have to take on a more kinaesthetic approach by getting involved in a practical activity. You need to get the most out of all learning opportunities.

Now try something different: mix it up a bit! Try another method of retaining information as shown in Activity 2.4.

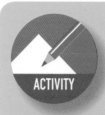

Activity 2.4

Look at the article by the Diversity Job Board (2012). How would you go about remembering the contents?

Cultural Diversity

All countries in the world have their own cultural heritage and identity, these can mean factors like their religious beliefs and language. In the modern world with the increase in air travel and also immigration due to population movement most countries now have small ethnic minority groups living with them. These groups will have their own culture and traditions, and it is this difference that can be said to provide cultural diversity to a country.

Nations where there is much cultural diversity can also sometimes be known as a multicultural society, this is the opposite of cultural uniformity. Diversity can take many different forms, for instance certain citizens may have their own dress style, food, language, traditions as well as different standards of morality.

The UK can be described as a truly diverse and multicultural country because of the immigration that has taken place there over the last fifty odd years. In these circumstances it has been the responsibility of successive UK governments to promote policies

(continued)

that encourage social cohesion and combat discrimination and inequality for all its citizens.

As you can see it is very important for race relations that all communities work together and have a sense of belonging and citizenship for the good of the country.

You should also note that diversity is not just limited to ethnicity but can also mean a indigenous persons background for instance their social class, sexual orientation as well as their gender.

In the UK there are a number of established main ethnic groups. The descendants of some of these are now third or fourth generation British citizens, the majority of whom have integrated well into mainstream British society.

Source: Diversity Job Board (2012).

OTHER STUDY METHODS

Today nursing courses can be taught using different teaching strategies, using traditional and non-traditional styles, such as attending lectures, seminars and tutorials, learning healthcare techniques at the bedside and attending workshops (see Chapter 1).

Other popular means of learning are distance or open learning, e-learning and multimedia approaches.

Distance Learning

Distance learning is usually where students are not physically present in a traditional classroom with a tutor present. Students work from written material, and video and audio recordings, and may meet infrequently with their tutor. An example of a provider of this approach is the Open University. Nursing updates also often use this approach, and are good for individuals with work commitments who are unable to travel to attend lectures or tutorials. The downside of the distant learning format is that if you don't understand something you may need to wait some time to get assistance.

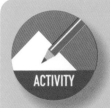

Activity 2.5

What are the advantages of study by distance learning? What are the disadvantages?

E-LEARNING

E-learning includes all forms of electronically supported learning and teaching. E-learning applications and processes include web-based learning, computer-based learning and virtual teaching. Delivery can be via the intranet, audio or video recordings, TV and CD-ROM. As a means of updating skills, many hospitals use e-learning packages for sessions, such as:

* waste management,
* fire safety theory,
* food hygiene,
* blood transfusion theory,
* calculations practice,
* medicines management,
* anaphylaxis,
* infection control,
* manual handling theory.

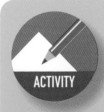

Activity 2.6

What are the advantages and disadvantages of e-learning?

TEST YOUR KNOWLEDGE

1   If you have concerns regarding your studies or personal issues affecting your course, what resource material would you refer to?

2   Below are questions from the paediatric and neonatal calculations test paper of a distance learning pack. See if you can answer the questions.

NOTE: without an explanation of how to do the calculations it may be quite difficult to complete. This is the downfall of distance learning, not being able to ask questions if you get stuck. All answers, showing full working out, are given in the Answers section at the back of the book.

You may use a calculator for the following calculations (although it is important to be able to work out the answer without a calculator). The following formulae may be useful.

Drug dosages for injection (and other liquid medications)

$$\text{Volume of drug to be given} = \frac{\text{What you want}}{\text{What you've got}} \times \text{volume}$$

This means the dose prescribed, divided by the dose you have available multiplied by the liquid amount.

Drugs according to body weight

$$\text{Correct dosage per day} = \text{weight (kg)} \times \text{does per kg}$$

Morphine formula

$$\text{Dose (mcg/kg per hour)} = \left[\left(\frac{\text{Amount (mg)} \times 1000}{50\text{mL}} \right) \Big/ \text{Weight} \right] \times \text{Rate infusion is prescribed at}$$

The amount in milligrams multiplied by by 1000 (to convert to micrograms/kg per hour), divided by 50 mL (of fluid in the syringe), then divide by the infant's weight, and multiply by the rate at which the infusion is prescribed.

Inotrope formula

$$\text{Dose (mcg/kg per minute)} = \frac{[(\frac{\text{Amount (mg)} \times 1000}{50mL})/\text{Weight}]}{60} \times \text{Rate infusion is prescribed at}$$

Amount (mg) × 1000 (to convert to micrograms/kg per hour), divided by 50 mL (of fluid in the syringe), then divide by the infant's weight, then divide by 60 to convert to per minute, multiplied by the rate at which the infusion is prescribed.

Inotrope examples include dopamine and dobutamine.

(a) Vancomycin is prescribed at 15 mg/kg BD. Baby weighs 975 g. What is the prescribed dose?

(b) Caffeine base is prescribed as 5 mg/kg per 24 hours to a baby weighing 1.8 kg. What amount of caffeine is prescribed?

(c) Benzylpenicillin IV is prescribed as 50 mg/kg. Baby weighs 4.2 kg.
  i What dose is prescribed?
  ii It comes as 600 mg in 4 mL of water. How much do you give?

(d) A baby weighing 2.2 kg is prescribed vitamin K at 0.4 mg/kg IM. What dose should be prescribed and how is it given?

(e) Paediatric IV digoxin comes as 50 micrograms/2 mL. The prescription is to

(continued)

administer 40 micrograms. What volume of digoxin would you administer?

(f) Morphine dose is calculated as 2 mg/kg for a concentrated solution.

  i A baby weighs 3.1 kg. How much morphine is prescribed?

  ii The pump is running at 0.5 mL/h. How many micrograms/kilogram per hour is the baby receiving? Use the morphine formula.

(g) Dopamine is calculated as 120 mg/kg for a concentrated solution.

  i Work out dose for the baby in question f (3.1 kg).

  ii The pump is running at 0.25 mL/h. How many micrograms/kilogram per minute is the baby receiving? Use the inotrope formula.

KEY POINTS

- Recognising patterns in text
- Establishing your own preferred learning style
- The VARK system of perception
- Distance learning
- E-learning

Bibliography

Boyd, C. (2013) *Calculation Skills for Nurses*. Wiley Blackwell, Oxford.

Diversity Job Board (2012) *Multicultural Britain*. www.diversityjobboard.co.uk.

Fleming, N. (2006) *Teaching and Learning Styles: VARK Strategies*. Fleming, Christchurch.

Gardiner, H. (1993) *Frames of Mind; the Theory of Multiple Intelligences*, 2nd edn. Fontana, London.

Honey, P. and Mumford, A. (1992) *The Manual of Learning Styles*. Peter Honey, Maidenhead.

Chapter 3

TAKING CONTROL

Study Skills for Nurses, First Edition. Claire Boyd and contributing author, Beverley Murray

Your success on your training course will not just be about intelligence – after all, you got to university, so you must be pretty bright – it is also about how you approach your studies and plan your time to meet your deadlines. As with all degrees, a degree in nursing takes a lot of hard work before reaching your graduation celebrations (Figure 3.1).

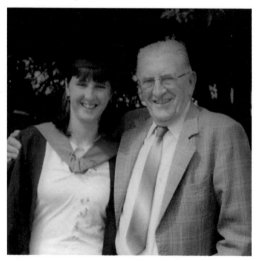

Figure 3.1 Graduation day

PLANNING

Studying in higher education requires you to plan your workload so that you can optimise your time effectively and maximise your productivity. When you first start at university, and receive information about your assignments, reports and case studies, and the maths tests you are required to pass, not to the mention competency assessments, you may feel somewhat overwhelmed by it all.

In the midst of this avalanche of work you will need to plan. It may seem like the straw that will break the camel's back: isn't it a waste of time spending what few hours you have left 'planning'? You will soon realise that the time you take to plan your workload will be well spent and *not* a waste. Get into the mindset of thinking that planning is not a luxury. It is a necessity that will make your studies more effective. Planning will also:

- help you to become more productive;
- enable you to stay focused: keeping your eye on the deadlines;
- help the quality of your work: not having to rush and produce less than your best;
- help to reduce your stress levels and stop panic setting in;
- enable you to see what has been done and what is left to do;
- help you to enjoy your course more, as you will not be in a state of fear throughout, and enable you to enjoy your leisure time more: you will have earned it;
- empower you: taking control of your studies, not them taking control of you.

PRIORITISING

You will often be given all your work at the start of a module and then you will need to make priorities. Obviously the closer deadlines will need to be worked on first, and any other important things. Do not make the mistake of starting work on a subject you enjoy most and pushing to the back those you may find harder. While working on an assignment you should continue reading and preparing for your classes and even making initial preparations for your other assignments.

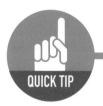

QUICK TIP

How to organise your study
- Use the planner at the back of this book to organise your shifts and study.
- Always try to complete your assignments a week ahead of the submission date.
- Always ask a tutor to review a first draft of assignments.
- Organise your priorities and stick to them: no distractions.
- Concentrate on the task in hand.
- Ask for help if you are struggling.
- Don't worry about perfection: just make sure you have met all the task criteria.
- Inform your mentor and tutor of any major crisis in your personal life and seek extensions if appropriate.

MANAGING YOUR WORK

One of the golden rules when managing your work is to use a planner and write down details of your workload. Look at the list of tasks and write down when you intend to do literature searches and reading, make notes, write, submit drafts, make improvements and hand in completed work. This procedure should be used on every piece of work you have been given. This is where your planner comes into play. Some people prefer to use a yearly planner, so that they can see the whole picture, with everything laid out in one go. But it is also a good idea just to jot down what you are doing on a week-to-week basis (see Test Your Knowledge at the end of this chapter).

ORGANISING YOURSELF

How you wish to organise yourself is up to you because what works well for one person may not work so well for someone else. You may wish to consider the following principles when organising your study plan.

- Prepare your study area well, with everything you need around you to suit your learning needs. Limit noise and distraction.
- Organise your study time in small chunks of 30 minutes or in much larger chunks (2, 4 or 6 hours, etc.), whichever suits you. Write this in your planner and take regular breaks.
- Organise your study time around the hours that suit you best (and around your clinical shift patterns): some people prefer the early morning and some prefer the dead of night to study. Set your alarm clock if you need to wake up early.
- Study skills experts often state that you should study after lectures, as your memory will be improved if you review your lecture notes straightaway rather than leaving them until much later.
- Don't spend hours and hours planning your schedule: some people make beautiful coloured charts when preparing their planner: there are more productive ways of spending your time! However, using colour to separate different tasks – deadline dates in red, literature searches in yellow, for instance – can be useful, giving you the information at a glance.
- Make sure you get enough sleep: nursing itself is very physical, and you will have your studies on top of this activity.
- Eat nutritious, well-balanced meals. Poor diet and lack of fluids can make you grouchy and tired. This can have an adverse effect on your motivation.
- Always over-estimate how long things are going to take (you may come across last minute problems). This way you will never run out of time to complete your assignments.
- Make the best use of the time you have: use a free evening to plan your essay; use an hour between lectures to visit the library; or use your journey to university to review your lecture notes.
- Don't forget to plan some time for relaxation and recreation. Sometimes it is important to step back (but not too far), as long as you are on target.

Students who have walked in your shoes offer the following advice.

Always try to complete your assignments a week ahead of the submission date.

Use the planner at the back of this book to organise your shifts and study.

Ask for help if you are struggling.

Don't worry about perfection: just make sure you have met all the task criteria.

Always ask a tutor to review a first draft of an assignment.

Inform your mentor and tutor of problems in your personal life and seek extensions if appropriate.

Organise your priorities and stick to them: no distractions (work before play).

QUICK TIP

WORKING IN GROUPS

Academic work usually focuses on the individual and their achievements in order to receive their degree. More emphasise is being now given to 'people skills': working with others to develop communication skills whilst working with others. In the healthcare profession, these people skills are vitally important. Throughout the Francis Report (Mid Staffordshire NHS Foundation Trust Public Inquiry 2013) looking at what went wrong in Mid Staffordshire

NHS Foundation Trust, many patients complained about the interpersonal skills of care staff.

Group work can take many forms, including seminars and/ or classroom activities, being taught clinical skills (at the bedside and in the classroom, discussion groups, support groups) and project assignments.

Group Project Assignments

If your assignment has been a project, the group may be asked to present their findings as a group also. When working in a group project, you will need to plan effectively in order to maximise efficiency and improve productivity.

Group working is an academic strategy as it enables the group to:

- share ideas and experiences;
- draw on members strengths and experiences;
- increase the quality of the output;
- strengthen problem-solving strategies;
- provide a supportive environment for challenging work;
- develop team-working skills;
- develop of interpersonal skills.

Ground rules

However, one of the first tasks to be decided upon by the group is the setting of *ground rules*, such as attending progress meetings and completing tasks allocated to you on time. This is where clear agendas and boundaries need to be established.

Once the ground rules have been established, start to look at the assignment.

Preparation around the subject

You will probably had had lectures and seminars on the assignment topic, so work co-operatively: read each other's notes, as your peers may have highlighted different points to you in their notes. It is important to establish a supportive group atmosphere.

Organise the task

Next, organise the task. Sit down and go through the assessment criteria and *discuss* what needs to be done to meet these criteria. During this planning stage you may disagree with ideas volunteered by other members of the group: this is fine as long as you do it in a non-critical way, suggesting improvements rather than being negative.

Listening to the group

It is important to listen to the whole group's ideas, allowing everyone to express their ideas. One person should not dominate these proceedings, but it is good to have one individual leading the process to avoid everyone shouting out at once and getting nowhere!

Group leader

The group may decide to rotate the role of chairperson. During the initial planning meeting it is important to ask questions to clarify anything you do not understand to avoid confusion later on.

Distribute tasks fairly

Once an agreement has been reached as to how the assignment will be approached, share out the work fairly, playing to each other's strengths. You will probably need to read around any area that has been allocated to you.

Follow-up meetings

Arrange regular meetings well in advance so that everyone can attend, to check how everyone is achieving their goals for the task.

When the group plans to meet again make sure that everyone has undertaken their agreed tasks. During subsequent meetings everyone needs to check that the group is on target. As the work progresses perhaps make links with each other's tasks, ready for blending your assignment should you be presenting your project to the larger group.

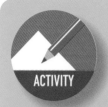

Activity 3.1

If the group encounters major difficulties, such as one member not having done work that needs to be presented soon to the whole class, or you feel that the group is not listening to you and you are being treated unfairly, what should you do?

PRESENTATION

A project assignment may mean that you have to present your project to a wider group and each person in the group should present what they have been working on. Many individuals feel very nervous about giving a presentation, but in nursing you may be asked to present research findings to a group of healthcare professionals or a topic for discussion at a job interview. Chapter 9 outlines the techniques used to give a presentation, but in general you should:

- make a few main points,
- use examples,
- speak clearly and slowly,
- repeat your main points and summarise what you have said.

If a group is presenting it is important to make all the joins seamless, with one talk flowing into the next. Otherwise individual talks by group members will seem very disjointed. They may even repeat each other: this is where the collaboration and teamwork are needed.

KNOWING WHEN TO STOP

Once you have achieved your task, be it planning, or completing a group task or individual assignment, you should know when to stop. Give yourself a pat on the back and move on. Time to get motivated for the next assignment. Sometimes we spend too long enjoying the glow of having achieved something and fall behind with future assignments. Equally, we may spend too much time tweaking the completed assignment: will you really gain higher marks with extra tinkering?

TEST YOUR KNOWLEDGE

Below is an outline weekly planner: produce your own and write in all your tasks for the next 4 weeks. Include time you intend to spend with support groups, conducting internet searches for assignments, meetings with your tutor, meetings with your mentor, preparing notes, typing up notes, etc., and, of course, any shifts you are working.

Month...	Monday	Tuesday	Wednesday	Thursday	Friday	Sat	Sun
Week 1							
Work shift							
Week 2							
Work shift							
Week 3							
Work shift							
Week 4							
Work shift							

An example of one week's completed planner is shown in the Answers section at the back of the book.

KEY POINTS

- Planning
- Prioritising
- Managing your work
- Organising yourself
- Working in groups

Bibliography

Mid Staffordshire NHS Foundation Trust Public Inquiry (2013) *Report of the Mid Staffordshire NHS Foundation Trust Public Inquiry; Executive Summary* (Chair: R. Francis). Stationery Office, London.

Northedge, A. (2005) *The Good Study Guide*. The Open University, Milton Keynes.

Chapter 4

INFORMATION SKILLS

Study Skills for Nurses, First Edition. Claire Boyd and contributing author, Beverley Murray

© 2014 John Wiley & Sons, Ltd. Published 2014 by John Wiley & Sons Ltd.

LEARNING OUTCOMES

By the end of this chapter you will have an understanding of library support, how to access various information resources and how to structure a question during a topic search.

FINDING INFORMATION

Imagine if searching for information was the same as going into a large shopping mall (the Internet). You wish to purchase a box of waterproof plasters (a journal article) which may take a lot of time – finding a shop that sells them, which floor they are located on, etc. – so you decide to visit a chemist's shop (bibliographic database) that only sells health-related items (journal articles). Here you discover that you can find the box of plasters (journal article) much more quickly.

Now for the real thing: the aim of searching for information is to discover or determine facts or accurate information about a topic. Healthcare students may at any time need to become proficient in undertaking information/literature searches to support them in areas such as:

- clinical practice,
- learning,
- continuous professional development,
- research.

Healthcare staff work in an environment that requires evidence-based practice so they need to be able to search and find information/literature with the aim of producing high-quality results.

When looking for information it is easy to get lost in the masses of documents and records that are available. It is all too easy to get hundreds of results, many of which are irrelevant, for example by entering a word or two into a search engine like Google.

IDENTIFYING AND SELECTING RELEVANT INFORMATION

You need to identify and evaluate sources effectively, as well as search efficiently for information/literature on any healthcare topic. This information can be accessed in various places, as explained below.

The Library

The library is most often the starting place for studying. When you join your university library you will find out about the range of services available and where you can get support on how to use library facilities and resources. Services provided by a library may include:

- electronic catalogues,
- bibliographic databases,
- books/e-books,
- journals/e-journals,
- a study area,
- access to photocopiers and scanners,
- a computer room,
- online library guides,
- Information skills training, e.g., literature searching

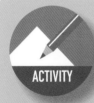

Activity 4.1

ACTIVITY

Go to your library.
- Check the classification scheme used to group books.
- Which class number applies to your subject?
- Find out how many items can you have on loan at once.
- For how long can you borrow books?
- Are there fines for late return of material?

Books

Books on a given subject are grouped together (classified) on the shelves. You can find the book's class number by looking it up in the library catalogue.

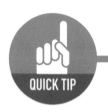

QUICK TIP

To find books it helps if you already know:

- **the author's surname and initials,**
- **the title of the book.**

Use your reading list to help you identify and select relevant information.

Use the latest information, for example the most up-to-date title and date of the latest edition of a book.

Journals

Journals contain the latest research on a subject as well as book reviews. Most journal articles have a short **abstract** at the beginning, which is a brief summary telling you what the article is about. Journals are published at regular intervals throughout the year, which can be weekly, bimonthly, monthly or quarterly. Each part is known as an **issue** and has a number. Journal issues/parts are collected into **volumes** which are also numbered, usually one for each year. The issue of *British Journal of Nursing* published on 10 May 2012 was volume 21, number 9. Volume 21 covers all the issues published in 2012.

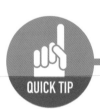

QUICK TIP

To find a journal article it helps if you already know:

- **the name of the journal,**
- **the title of the article,**
- **the year the article was published, and the volume and issue number,**
- **the name and initials of the article's author(s).**

Evidence-Based Sources

The term **evidence-based source** can apply to any of the
following types of source.

- **Primary** source: this refers to first-hand, primary
  research that is based upon questionnaires,
  observations or experiments. It is published in research
  articles in journals.
- **Secondary** source, or second-hand source: this
  is where another source is created from previous
  evidence or studies. Some common secondary
  sources are:
  - The **Cochrane Library** (www.thecochranelibrary.
    com), which publishes systematic reviews based on
    a particular research question. Research evidence
    from the primary literature is selected, combined
    and appraised to produce a comprehensive review
    of the latest evidence in the field.
  - Clinical guidelines, for example NICE, NICE
    Evidence (www.evidence.nhs.uk, www.nice.org.uk/)
  - Journals of secondary publication, such as
    Evidence Based Nursing (EBN; ebn.bmj.com).

The Internet

The internet began in the 1950s with the development of
computers.

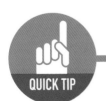

QUICK TIP

**Although you may be tempted to rely
on direct internet searching for finding
information it is worth remembering
that:**

- **internet search engines look for words
  or word combinations anywhere on the
  web page regardless of relevance,**
- **websites can be created without being
  checked or authenticated, so may be of
  dubious value.**

Bibliographic Healthcare Databases

Bibliographic healthcare databases allow you to search and locate primary research (journal articles). Your library will subscribe to various databases and can provide you with information on how to access them together with training in how to search for literature.

HOW TO SEARCH BIBLIOGRAPHIC DATABASES EFFECTIVELY

Search Strategy

To overcome the problem of retrieving unwanted results it is worth taking a few minutes before you start to think about what exactly you are looking for and to focus your question.

Breaking Your Topic into Concepts

When thinking about your topic, it is useful to break it down into two, three or four concepts (depending on the information you are looking for) and then choose the most pertinent concepts to search for.

Building Your Question

Once you have decided on your concepts you can use them to create a well-structured question. The PICO framework can be useful: PICO stands for Patient/Population, Intervention or exposure, Comparisons, Outcome (Figure 4.1). Appendix 1, at the back of this book, shows alternative question frameworks.

Looking at Your Concepts

Once you have established the concepts in your question you need to identify the **key words** for each concept that you can use in your search. You need to think about

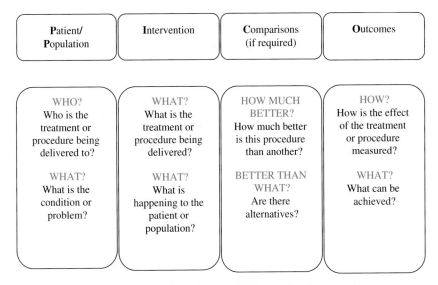

Figure 4.1 The main concepts for using the PICO question framework

synonyms and alternative terms for the subject you are interested in.

	Search term	Synonyms
P	stroke(s)	cerebrovascular accident
I	warfarin	warfarin sodium
C	dietary advice	diet, nutrition
O	risk of further strokes reduced	risk reduction

Also think about variations in word endings. **Truncating** your term will allow for variations in word endings, which means that you do not have to carry out several separate searches. The truncation symbol is often an asterisk (*) and is used as a substitute for zero or more characters. So searching for alcohol* will find instances of *alcohol, alcoholic, alcoholics* and alcoholism.

Different spellings also need to be considered. **Wildcard** searches allow you to search for spelling variations, as might be found in research produced in countries that use US English. The symbol is often a question mark (?), and is used as a substitute for zero or one character. So searching for *leuk?emia* retrieves both *leukaemia* and *leukemia*.

Carrying Out an Effective Search

Once you have broken your search question into its concepts and thought about alternative terms for each concept you are ready to choose a resource in which to search for information. For example, this can involve choosing to search in a **bibliographic database**. These databases index publications on a given subject, then list and reference them, allowing users to conduct literature searches. Key databases include:

- CINAHL (Cumulative Index of Nursing and Allied Health Literature),
- Medline,
- Embase,
- PsycINFO,
- AMED.

Searching a 'Free-Text' Database

Different databases are searched in different ways. Each will have instructions and give help on how to enter your search terms. You can search a database such as CINAHL by entering key word(s) in the search box and clicking **Search**.

Key words can be searched for in different parts, or **search fields**, of an article. These will include **title and abstract**, **author**, **ISSN number**, **journal name**, **publication type**, **title** and **any field**. The default option may be to search for key words in the title and abstract, so be sure to check before starting.

QUICK TIP

Quotation marks or brackets may be used around phrases and numbers, for example "heart attack" or "diabetes type 2", to keep the words together in that exact phrase. This way, only articles containing (for example) the single phrase *heart attack* will be found; those with *heart* but not *attack* will not be listed in your search results, and neither will those containing both words but which do not occur together. This allows you to ignore irrelevant articles. Check the database for examples of how to do this, as single or double quotation marks may be used.

Using operators (Boolean searching)

Once you have decided on your search terms and alternative terms you can combine them using Boolean operators. These allow you to combine, include and exclude. In this way can combine the results for each alternative term that you used in each concept so that you get a set of results that contains one or other term, both or all of them.

The Boolean operators **AND**, **OR** and **NOT** allow you to combine your searches to produce the most relevant set of results.

- AND combines two terms or searches together, finding any articles which contain both. This makes a search more specific, so you will end up with fewer results. For example, searching for **"heart attack" AND aspirin** will find articles that contain both terms.
- OR retrieves any articles which contain one or other (or both) of the terms you search for. It is useful for broadening out a search, and you will end up with more results. For example, searching for **"myocardial**

infarction" **OR** "**heart attack**" will find articles that
contain one or other, or both, of these terms.

- NOT excludes any record that contains an unwanted
term. This narrows down a search. For example,
"**myocardial infarction**" **NOT** "**heart attack**" will
show you all the results containing only *myocardial
infarction*. Similarly searching for "**myocardial
infarction**" **NOT** "**beta-blockers**" will find any articles
mentioning *myocardial infarction* except those that
mention *beta-blockers*.

- AND, OR and NOT can be used together in various
combinations to retrieve a very specific set of
records.

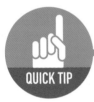

QUICK TIP

**AND/NOT refining, exclusive
OR broadening, inclusive**

Searching a Database with a Thesaurus

A database **thesaurus** is an index or list of the preferred
subject headings (other **search terms**) you can use to search
the database. A thesaurus is useful because it:

- lists the preferred search terms used by the database,
- suggests related terms and broader or narrower
subject headings.

Use the thesaurus to find the appropriate thesaurus term(s)
to match your search term(s) and select one or more.

Select the appropriate Boolean operators to combine terms
from the thesaurus that you want to search, such as **cancer
OR neoplasm** and **cancer NOT neoplasm**.

Limiting your Search

If you have more references than you expected there are
several ways to refine your search to make them more

relevant. Limiting functions allow you to restrict your search in various ways. An example list of a database's limits could be:

- date (specifying a range of publication years),
- article type (e.g. abstracts, references available),
- publication types (e.g. research articles, reviews),
- whether studies were conducted on humans or animals,
- gender,
- age groups,
- language,
- other.

Viewing and reviewing the results of your search

The results can be viewed and there may be a link to the full text of an article from the database, linking to an e-journal that the library subscribes to. You may also have to manually search the library catalogue to see if the library holds copies of the print journals (volume/issue) listed in your search results.

QUICK TIP

Review your references throughout your search to make sure that your results continue to be relevant and appropriate.

Author Searching

You can construct a search to retrieve articles by particular authors by changing the search option from the default (e.g. Title/Abstract) to Author.

Journal Searching

Similarly you can search by journal name by keying in the journal title. You will need to follow the database's instructions on how to enter your search terms; remember that not all databases are the same.

You can combine **Author** and **Journal name** search lines with topic searches if this is appropriate for the information you wish to retrieve.

Here's a summary of how to find and search in the literature.

- Search key words in a selected bibliographic database e.g. CINAHL.
- Consider time scale, for example going back only 5 years.
- Enter key words for each search and click Search.

QUICK TIP

Contact the library for help with your searches.

TEST YOUR KNOWLEDGE

1 What does PICO stand for?
2 Bibliographic databases search for keywords in which parts of an article?
3 What limits can be selected for your search?
4 When would you use quotation marks in your search term?
5 Truncating your term will …?
6 Wildcards allow you to …?
7 What are the three Boolean operators?
8 Which operators make a search more specific (with fewer results)?
9 Which operator broadens out a search (with more results)?
10 Can you search to retrieve articles by certain authors or by journal name?

KEY POINTS

- Finding information
- Evidence-based sources
- Searching effectively

Bibliography

Davies, K.S. (2011) Formulating the evidence based practice question: a review of the frameworks. *Evidence Based Library and Information Practice* 6(2), 75–80.

Doyle, L. et al. (2009) An overview of mixed methods research. *Journal of Research in Nursing* 14(2), 175–185.

Strauss, S.E., Glasziou, P., Richardson, W.S. and Haynes, R.B. (2011) *Evidence-Based Medicine: How to Practice and Teach It*, 4th edn. Churchill Livingstone, London; Appendix: Glossary pp. 269–273.

Chapter 5

READING EFFECTIVELY

Study Skills for Nurses, First Edition. Claire Boyd and contributing author, Beverley Murray
© 2014 John Wiley & Sons, Ltd. Published 2014 by John Wiley & Sons Ltd.

LEARNING OUTCOMES

By the end of this chapter you will have an understanding of the general principles of reading effectively, including active reading, speed reading, spellchecking your work and critical reading skills.

Let's start with a two minute test: see Activity 5.1.

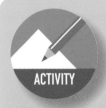

Activity 5.1

Two minute test

1 Read everything before you do anything.
2 Put your initials in the upper left-hand corner of this page.
3 Circle the word 'page' on the second task.
4 Draw five small circles in the upper-right hand corner of the page.
5 Put an X in each circle mentioned in task 4.
6 Draw a square around each circle.
7 Sign your name under 'Chapter 5' on this page.
8 After 'Reading Effectively' write 'yes' three times.
9 Put a circle around task numbers 2 and 7.
10 Put an X in the lower right-hand corner of the page.
11 Draw a triangle around the X you have just made.
12 Multiply 50 by 20.
13 Draw a circle around the word 'page' in task 4.
14 On the reverse side of this page, add 105 and 439.
15 Put a circle around your answer to this problem.
16 Put three small dots with your pen or pencil here.
17 Now you have finished reading carefully, do only tasks 1 and 2.

OK did you miss the point of Activity 5.1? This was obviously just a bit of fun, but reading effectively is not just about reading research articles correctly. There are also more far-reaching considerations, such as when reading exam questions or prescription charts. We can't afford to misread what is in front of us.

READING FASTER

The ability to read *quickly but effectively* is not the answer to every problem, but if you have a good reading speed you will be able to skim and scan more quickly, saving yourself valuable time.

NOTE: for texts with condensed information, detailed instructions, formulae and equations, *slow* reading may be more beneficial (see later).

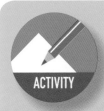

Activity 5.2

ACTIVITY

Read the passage at the speed you would normally read a newspaper. Time yourself with a stopwatch or a watch with a second hand.

DEMENTIA

Dementia is a physical disease process, used to describe a set of symptoms that occur when the brain is damaged by specific diseases causing a progressive deterioration of brain tissue, increased death of nerve cells and loss of function.

There are approximately 70 disorders which cause dementia, but the four main types are:

- Alzheimer's disease,
- vascular dementia,
- lewy body dementia,
- fronto-temporal dementia.

(continued)

Alzheimer's Disease

There is an accumulation of abnormal amyloid between nerve cells (neurons) in the brain. There is also abnormal tau protein found as 'tangles' inside the neurons.

Early onset or familial Alzheimer's is often linked to genetic mutations, but most cases of Alzheimer's dementia are not genetic or inherited.

Vascular Dementia

Vascular dementia occurs because of small blood vessel disease to 25% of the brain, including microscopic bleeding and blood vessel blockage.

Vascular dementia is commonly recognised as a mixed diagnosis with Alzheimer's disease. Depending where the brain injury has occurred, determines how the individual's thinking and physical functions are affected.

Lewy Body Dementia

Lewy bodies are tiny spherical abnormal protein deposits found in the cortex and substantia nigra within the brain. Their presence disrupts the brain's normal functioning by interrupting the action of chemical messengers, such as acetylcholine and dopamine.

People with LBD may experience physical impairments similar to those found in Parkinson's disease. They may also experience very vivid visual hallucinations.

Fronto-Temporal Dementia

The term fronto-temporal dementia covers a range of conditions, such as Pick's disease, caused by damage to the frontal lobe and/or the temporal parts of the brain. These areas of the brain are responsible for our emotional responses, language skills and behaviour.

There are currently no medications available which 'treat' the cause of dementia, but there are a number of medications which can help improve some of the symptoms in Alzheimer's and lewy body dementia:

- donepezil (Aricept),
- rivastigmine (Exelon),
- galantamine (Reminyl),
- memantine (Ebixa).

Now work out your reading speed.

Time to read = ... seconds

The passage is approximately 311 words long, so use the following calculation.

$$\frac{311 \times 60}{\text{Reading time (seconds)}} = \frac{18\,660}{\text{Reading time (seconds)}}$$
$$= \text{No. of words/minute}$$

For example, if you took 60 seconds to read the article, your reading speed would be:

$$\frac{18\,660}{60 \text{ seconds}} = 311 \text{ words per minute}$$

OK, so it's nice to know your reading speed, but what does it mean in reality? If you read the passage at a speed of:

- 240 words per minute or more, your reading speed is good.
- less than 240 words per minute, then you will benefit from more practice at speed reading.

When you are studying and time is very precious, speed reading can really save you time. Two forms of speed reading are described here.

- **Scanning:** this is where you scan parts of the text, perhaps just looking at the first and last paragraphs, introductions and conclusions. You can then stop at the really important information to read this more fully.
- **Skimming:** this is where you skip over the details, just getting the gist of the book or article. By skimming over the text we can establish whether the text is going to be any good to us, thus saving us time.

Detailed Reading

Detailed reading is when we need to extract all the information in order to learn from the text, perhaps when we are revising for an exam. You need to read every word. Perhaps you will chose to scan or skim first, before going back to read the finer points of the text.

If at any point you are unsure what a word or phase means you will need to stop to look it up in a dictionary before moving on. This method of reading – non-passive – is also known as **active reading**.

ACTIVE READING

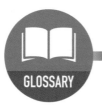

Connective tissue
Material between the cells of the body that gives tissues form and strength.

Activity 5.3

The text here shows the different types of connective tissue found in the body. Read and learn.

CONNECTIVE TISSUE

Connective tissue is the most abundant tissue in the body, its cells are more widely separated than epithelium and there are large amounts of intercellular material present. It may contain fibres of matrix, be dense or rigid, or of a semi-solid jelly like consistency or liquid. It has a mechanical function and connects different tissue types together e.g. muscles and bones. Its function is for protection, insulation, transport, support and binding.

There are eight types of connective tissue which you will find as you learn the body systems will link into this explanation.

1 **Areolar tissue:** this is the most general connective tissue in the human body.
   Structure: it is elastic, allowing a high degree of relative movement and has reticular fibres interspersed with numerous connective tissue cells in a semi-solid permeable matrix which allows fluids to pass through it.

   Function: found all over the body connecting and supporting other tissues e.g. it binds skin to muscles

   Location: between skin and muscles, supporting blood vessels and nerves, in the alimentary canal.

2 **Adipose tissue,** also known as fatty tissue. Food which is excess to requirements is converted into fat and stored in adipose cells; up to 25% of the body weight of a well-fed adult is white adipose tissue. There are also small quantities of brown adipose tissue which differs in that it has a more extensive network of capillaries than white. Metabolised brown adipose tissue produces more heat and less energy than white.

   Structure: made up of large amounts of fat cells with a matrix of areolar tissue.

(continued)

Function: white: support, protection and insulation, and it is also a food reserve; brown: it helps retain heat as it is a poor conductor of heat, and it is also an energy store.

Location: white: eyes, kidneys, between muscles and under the skin; brown, walls of large blood vessels, trunk, nape of neck, between the scapulae.

3 Lymphoid tissue

Structure: semi-solid tissue; has some white fibres but these are not in bundles.

Function: lymphocyte cells, of which there are many, have a disease control function – they engulf and destroy bacteria.

Location: found in lymph nodes, thymus, the spleen, the tonsils, the wall of the large intestine, the appendix and the glands of the small intestine.

4 Yellow elastic tissue

Structure: mainly composed of elastic fibres and very few cells; this tissue is capable of considerable extension and recoil.

Function: to enable stretch and recoil of organs and vessels.

Location: in areas such as trachea, bronchi, lung tissue, the large arteries, the stomach and bladder.

5 White fibrous tissue

Structure: a strong connective tissue but with little elasticity. Closed packed bundles of collagen fibres with a few cells in rows beneath the fibres. The fibres all run in the same direction.

Function: connection and protection of parts of the body.

Location: the periosteum of bone; forms ligaments, the facia of muscles and tendons; forms the outer protection of some organs e.g. around the kidneys, the dura of the brain.

6 Bone, osseous tissue: next to the teeth bone is the hardest tissue in the body.

Structure: 25% water, 30% organic material, 45% inorganic salts.

Function: to support and protect the body and all its organs. To produce blood cells in the bone marrow. There are two types: compact, which is dense bone for strength; cancellous, for structure bearing and cellular development.

Location: the skeletal structure.

7 Vascular tissue (blood): this is a connective tissue.
Structure: contains 45% cells – erythrocytes (red blood cells), leucocytes (white blood cells), thrombocytes (platelets) – and 55% plasma.

Function: to transport oxygen and food to all the cells of the body (erythrocytes), to fight infection (leucocytes) and to clot (thrombocytes).

8 Hyaline cartilage: the most common type of cartilage, particularly resilient.
Structure: bluish white elastic substance of chondrocyte cells which are grouped together in a solid matrix which is embedded fine collagen fibrils.

Function: protection, provides flexibility, support and aids movement of joints.

Location: forms costal cartilages (connect ribs to sternum), parts of larynx, trachea and bronchi, nose and end of bones which form joints.

a Hyaline yellow elastic cartilage
Structure: it has elastic fibres distributed in the solid matrix.

Function: flexibility, maintains shape, gives support.

Location: found in parts of the body that move freely: the pinnae (cartilage part of the ear), part of the wall of blood vessels, Eustachian tubes (inner ear), epiglottis.

(continued)

b **Hyaline white fibrocartilage**

Structure: tough bundle of dense white fibres in the matrix, similar to hyaline cartilage with widely dispersed cells and is slightly flexible tissue.

Function: to absorb shock.

Location: it is the discs between the vertebrae, the pad between the knee joint bones, found in the hip, shoulder sockets and the pubic symphysis.

As you were asked to learn the contents of this text, you should have used your active reading skills. Be honest with yourself, did you look at it, read the words and then, when finished, realise that you had not actually taken anything in? It does not help matters if the typeface is hard to read and very small. You thought you were concentrating, but now looking back at what you have just read, you may find that you cannot really remember much of the contents. This does not mean that you cannot concentrate, cannot read properly or even that you have any difficulty at recalling information. It happens to everybody. This activity also shows that reading should only be undertaken when you are alert and in the right frame of mind to do so. It is no good forcing yourself to read when your head is buzzing with other things, as this will just waste your time as you will not be actively reading.

It is very common for the reader's mind to go into neutral as early as 30 seconds after starting to read a textbook, let alone a boring piece of information on connective tissue. This loss of concentration usually happens when you sit down with no other reason for reading than the thought, 'I really must read some more of this…'.

The problem is caused by not reading *actively*. But being active when reading does not just happen, it has to be planned. **SQ3R** is a simple method of planning your reading so that it is more active, more purposeful and much more productive (see Box 5.1).

Box 5.1

SQ3R stands for:

Survey, Question, Read, Recall, Review

Survey

Have a quick look through the book, chapter or article to see what it is about and what you can expect to get out of it. You may also find it helpful to survey the list of contents and the index.

Question

Write down the questions you will be able to answer when you have read the book (or chapter or article) properly. The survey you have just done and your own needs will help you to formulate the questions.

Read

Once you have some useful questions, reading is easy. All you have to do is find where the answers to your questions are and read those bits carefully, perhaps making a few notes, sketching one or two diagrams, doing some calculations to make sure you understand them, and so on. Once you have the information you need, stop reading.

Recall

Try to answer all the questions without looking at the book or your notes. You will soon find out what you have learned and what you need to spend more time on.

Review

Go back to the book to check that your answers are right. Go over the things you have got wrong or could not answer.

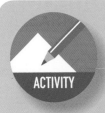

Activity 5.4

Now look at the questions below and read the connective tissue text again.

1   How many types of hyaline cartilage did the text list?
2   Where in the body can yellow elastic connective tissue be found?
3   What is the function of vascular tissue?
4   What is the structure of blood?

Keeping focused, perhaps by only looking at the questions you needed to answer, has helped your recall and saved you time.

TIPS FOR LEARNING

Other techniques of helping you with your Active reading is by underlining or **highlighting** key points in the text. You may also wish to note key words. Also, writing summaries and/or spider diagrams (see Chapter 6) and putting the information into tables can help you to retain information from active reading.

NOTE: you should not highlight, underline or make notes in borrowed books.

From the information on connective tissue that is presented in a very dry format and non-user-friendly typeface, we can produce a more visual depiction of the eight types of connective tissue (see Figure 5.1).

Now if I asked you to name the eight types of connective tissue from this visual interpretation then active learning may have taken place, especially for the visual learners among us.

Studying at an academic level involves using techniques to facilitate learning, such as speed reading and active reading. Now you know the strategies it is important to practise these skills to become proficient.

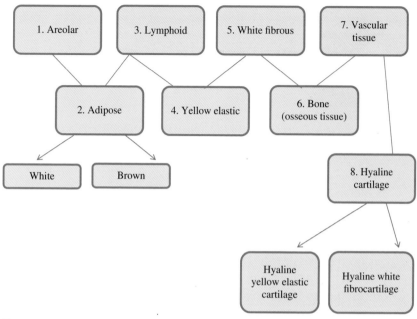

Figure 5.1 Eight types of connective tissue

CHECKING YOUR WORK

Before submitting your work you need to check it for spelling, punctuation and layout to iron out any mistakes. This is sometimes called 'proof reading'. It is also the last check to make sure that you have indeed answered the assignment question or met the report brief. It goes without saying that checking your work before submission is vital to receiving good grades throughout your course. However, checking is an acquired skill. It is often difficult to spot your own mistakes, as your brain may tell you what you *should* be seeing rather than what is actually written on the paper!

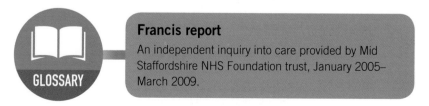

GLOSSARY

Francis report

An independent inquiry into care provided by Mid Staffordshire NHS Foundation trust, January 2005– March 2009.

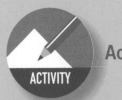

Activity 5.5

Below is part of a student's psychology essay. Can you spot any errors?

Individual's may infer attributes to whole groups of people, known as 'sterotyping' which is, according to Tagiuri (1969) (as cited by Gross 1994, p. 482) categorising people into identifiable groups and attributing to them qualities believed to be typical to members of that group. In nursing profession, media imagery of stereotypes has been endlessly reiterated in films, television and literature, which in turn may influence the general public's image of the nurse: Hudson-Jones (1989) gives a personel reflection that there are six major catogories: "Angel of Mercy, Handmaiden to the Physician, Woman in White, Sex Symbol/Idiot, Battle-Axe, Torturer" (Hudson-Jones 1989, p. 211).

However, members of the general pubic may disagree with Hudson-Jones in his opinion of only six stereotypes, perhaps having a 'nursing stereotype' of their own, especially in light of recent press reports around the lapses in care (Dreaper 2012), and lack of compassion patients have been recieving (Royal College of Nursing 2010) coupled with the Francis Report (Mid Staffordshire NHS Foundation Trust Public Inquiry 2013).

'Labelling' individuals into a stereotypical role can be extremely problamatic due to the fact that they take little or no account of the uniqueness and individuality of humans in general.

How many errors did you spot?

0–6 Your checking skills need improving
7–9 Not bad checking skills, but you still have room for improvement
10 Excellent checking skills

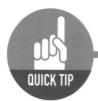

QUICK TIP

Get a friend or peer to check your work before submitting. They might notice mistakes you have missed.

To emphasise the importance of checking your written work, below are examples of mistakes found in patient medical notes, showing that the medical secretary had not read what was typed, or that the medic had not properly thought through what they were dictating.

- Patient's medical history has been remarkably insignificant with only a 40 pound weight gain in the past 3 days.
- She has no rigors or shaking chills, but her husband states that she was very hot in bed last night.
- On the second day, the knee was better and on the third day it had disappeared.
- The patient is tearful and crying constantly. She also appears to be depressed.
- The patient has been depressed since she began seeing me in 1993, much too long.
- Discharge status: alive, but without my permission.
- Healthy appearing decrepit 69-year-old male, mentally alert, but forgetful.
- She is numb from her toes down.
- While in ER, she was examined, X-rated and sent home.
- The skin was moist and dry.
- Occasional, constant infrequent headaches.
- Patient was alert and unresponsive.
- Rectal examination revealed a normal size thyroid.
- She stated that she had been constipated for most of her life until she got a divorce.
- Both breasts are equal and reactive to light and accommodation.
- Examination of genitalia reveals that he is circus sized and big too.
- Skin: somewhat pale, but present.
- Large brown stool ambulating in the hall, best sample yet.

- Patient has two teenage children, but no other abnormalities.
- When she fainted, her eyes rolled around the room.
- The patient was in his usual state of good health until his aeroplane ran out of fuel and crashed.
- Between you and me, we ought to get this lady pregnant pretty easy I'd say.
- She slipped on the ice and apparently her legs went in separate directions in early December.

Source: Lederer (2002).

CRITICAL READING

Imagine if critical/analytical reading was like a court of law and the journal article is the (defendant). You are the prosecutor who makes a cross-examination when analysing the article. You ask questions to verify whether the article is 'telling the truth' or not (defendant is 'guilty'). You are also the defence by reading/analysing the article to find the evidence in the article that confirms it is telling the truth or that the article (defendant) is 'not guilty'.

When reading a scientific paper/journal article you need to judge and question its scientific worth by approaching it in a structured way in order to identify and evaluate the important elements.

Select a Topic/Question

A research question asks the following.

- What is happening? (e.g. what is the effectiveness of a treatment?)
- How does it happen? (e.g. what is the mechanism of a treatment?)
- For whom and why does it happen?

Published research

A research question may be answered using data in the form of words (**qualitative research**), numbers (**quantitative research**) or a combination of both (**mixed-methods research**) (Figure 5.2).

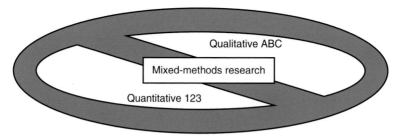

Figure 5.2 Published research

Qualitative research (inductive)

Qualitative research is 'used to explore and understand people's beliefs, attitudes, experiences, behaviour and interactions' (Bandolier, www.medicine.ox.ac.uk/bandolier/booth/glossary/qualres.html). Qualitative research often uses an **inductive** research strategy which aims to explore, describe and interpret the subject matter. This can lead to the development of theories (e.g. nursing theory) which can then be tested or to the development of questionnaires which aim to quantify important factors.

Quantitative research (deductive)

This type of research '…generates numerical data or data that can be converted into numbers, for example clinical trials…' (www.medicine.ox.ac.uk/bandolier/booth/glossary/qualres.html).

Mixed-methods research

Mixed-methods research is a methodology for conducting research that involves collecting, analysing and integrating (or mixing) quantitative and qualitative research (and data) in a single study. Its purpose is that both qualitative and quantitative research in combination provide a better understanding of a research problem or issue than either research approach alone (www.nd.edu.au/downloads/research/ihrr/using_mixed_methods_approach_to_enhance_and_validate_your_research.pdf).

Search Appropriate Sources

Sources and levels of evidence are shown in Figure 5.3, and they are defined in the glossary in Appendix 2 (see the back

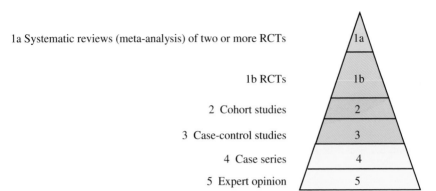

1a Systematic reviews (meta-analysis) of two or more RCTs

1b RCTs

2 Cohort studies

3 Case-control studies

4 Case series

5 Expert opinion

Figure 5.3 Sources of evidence. RCT, randomized controlled trial

of this book). See also Chapter 4 on evidence-based sources (primary and secondary). One way to evaluate literature relating to efficacy and effectiveness of a treatment is the hierarchical approach. It has strengths and weaknesses but is widely used.

Reading Critically

Do you read an article or do you *read* so as to *analyse/ evaluate* the article to decide if it is valid, genuine, useful, 'telling the truth?'

What is a critical reading?

You will not read everything during your studies in a critical or in-depth manner: what you read and your purpose will affect the way you read. This chapter is concerned with **primary sources** – journal articles – and how to evaluate them.

Critical reading is/should be:

- systematic, utilising a framework or 'tool',
- objective, basing judgements on careful analysis of the facts, not on personal opinions,
- thorough, not skipping the difficult bits,
- underpinned by theoretical understanding.

Critical reading is not:

- just an assessment of results,
- all about statistical analysis,
- just the 'easy' bits (introduction, results and conclusion).

Critical reading is good practice and necessary for evidence-based material. It gets easier and quicker with practice.

Why is critical reading important?

Critical reading is vital to **evidence-based practice** (EBP) and you need to be able to assess whether the information contained in the sources you find is accurate and whether the results presented are reliable. You need to show that you have read, understood and evaluated the relevant information for your chosen topic/question. Figure 5.4 gives the five stages of the EBP process.

Critical reading supports sound decision making based on the best available evidence, and helps to determine the three Rs:

- how **rigorous** a piece of research is,
- what the **results** are telling us,
- how **relevant** it is to the patient.

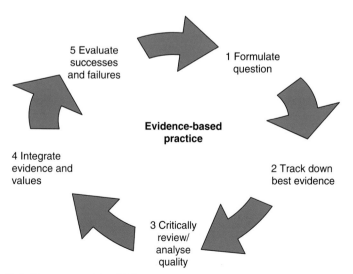

5 Evaluate successes and failures

1 Formulate question

Evidence-based practice

4 Integrate evidence and values

2 Track down best evidence

3 Critically review/ analyse quality

Figure 5.4 Five stages of the EBP process

How to Read Critically or What to Look For

Title Clear and succinct summary of what the paper is about?

Authors/date Author details? (place of work, etc.)

Introduction Logical and knowledgeable? An up-to-date view? Why was the work carried out?

Methods How was the work done? Are all relevant details of the procedure included? How were the data analysed?

Results How precise are the results? How are they presented? How readily can they be understood?

Discussion How does the author interpret the results in relation to the question posed in the introduction?

Conclusion Justified and valid? Does it answer the question?

Skills/Help to Read Critically

Comprehension Ask critical questions to help you to understand what the main point of a paper is and what the author is saying.

- **Comparison** Compare or relate the paper to other work in the field and to other papers on the same topic.
- **Interpretation** Check that the conclusions follow from the results: do you agree? Do you have a different view?
- **Analysis** Do you think/agree the evidence supports the argument? (See Appendix 3.)
- **Evaluation** Does the author estimate or assume the conclusion from the results? Is this paper good practice?

NOTE: remember! Evidence-based practice (EBP).

APPRAISING WEBSITES

Anybody can put anything on the internet so, when you are appraising information obtained from a website, bear in mind the following things.

- Website address: .org, .ac.uk, .gov are better than .co.uk and .com (see Quick Tip below)

- Content: who is the intended audience? What is the purpose of the site? How accurate is it? Are the sources of external information provided/cited?
- Source: who is/are the author(s)? Is it current (up to date)? Depth/breadth of coverage, bias? Are there any conflicts of interest (e.g. sponsorship)?
- Structure: graphics, presentation, grammar or spelling errors, ease of use?

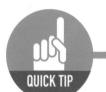

QUICK TIP

You can identify the source of a website by the ending of the address.

www...ac.uk or .edu	**Academic institution/ university**
www...gov.uk	**Government department**
www...org.uk	**Non-profit organisation or charity**
www...co.uk or .com	**Commercial company**
www...nhs.uk	**NHS organisation**

CRITICAL APPRAISAL

Critical appraisal (or CASP) is 'The process of assessing and interpreting evidence by systematically considering its validity, results and relevance' (www.medicine.ox.ac.uk/bandolier/booth/glossary/critapp.htm).

There are appraisal tools for:

- systematic reviews,
- randomised controlled trials,
- qualitative research studies,
- economic evaluation studies,
- cohort studies,
- case-control studies,
- diagnostic test studies,

You can download these tools to assist you in appraising and evaluating each article that you read depending on the research type. Often the type of research can be found in the title (e.g. What proportion of patients...: a systematic review).

CASP tools help you to appraise articles by providing questions regarding validity and by giving hints as to what to look for in the text of the article. For a CASP resource see the Website section at the end of the chapter.

TEST YOUR KNOWLEDGE

Now let's put your newly acquired skills to the test.

1 What is active reading?
2 What does SQ3R stand for?
3 Read the connective tissue text (Activity 5.3) again and put the information into a table.
4 Proof read this paragraph:

> Thorndike (1920) found that individuals have a tendency to be 'generous' in their impressions of others if given a description of that person containing one or two positive traits, known as the Halo effect. For example, if an individual is described as being intelligent and having a good sense of humour, and a positive impression is formed of that individual, other favourable attributes may then be further applied to that individual (perhaps inaccurately). The Halo effect may also be applied in the negative.

5 Name two types of research.
6 What skills are needed to read critically?

KEY POINTS

- Speed reading
- Active reading
- Using the SQ3R technique
- Checking your work
- Critical reading

Bibliography

Burns. N. and Grove, S.K. (2005) *The Practice of Nursing Research: Conduct, Critique, and Utilization*, 5th edn. Elsevier Saunders, St. Louis, MO.

Dreaper, J. (2012) Campaign to show 'skill and compassion' of nurses. BBC News, Health, 17 September.

Gross, R. (1994) *Psychology – The Science of Mind and Behaviour*, 2nd edn. Hodder and Stoughton, London.

Hudson-Jones, J. (1989) *Images of Nurses – Perspective from History, Art and Literature*. University of Pennsylvania, Philadelphia.

Lederer, R. (2002) *The Bride of Anguished English*. Griffin, New York.

Mid Staffordshire NHS Foundation Trust Public Inquiry (2013) *Report of the Mid Staffordshire NHS Foundation Trust Public Inquiry; Executive Summary* (Chair: R. Francis). Stationery Office, London.

Royal College of Nursing (2010) *The Principles of Nursing Practice*. Royal College of Nursing, London. www.rcn.org.uk/publications

Thorndike, E.L. (1920) A constant error in psychological ratings. *Journal of Applied Psychology* 4(1), 25–29.

Website

CASP UK, www.casp-uk.net/

Chapter 6

MAKING NOTES

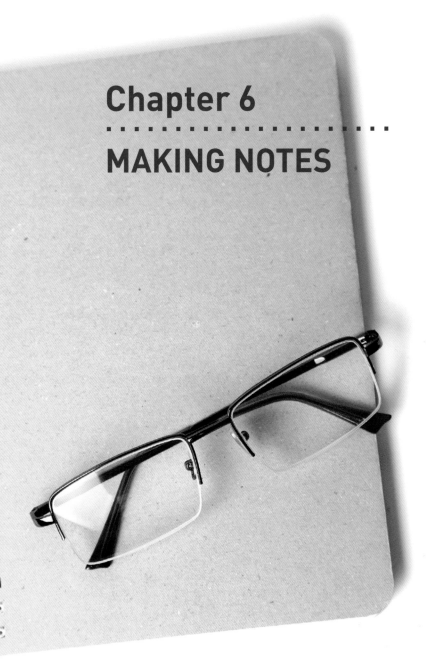

Study Skills for Nurses, First Edition. Claire Boyd and contributing author, Beverley Murray
© 2014 John Wiley & Sons, Ltd. Published 2014 by John Wiley & Sons Ltd.

LEARNING OUTCOMES

By the end of this chapter you will have an understanding of the value of note-taking during academic study and will have learned some effective note-taking strategies.

Note-taking is a skill: many of us take vast quantities of notes from lectures or articles and never look at them again due to the fast pace of our academic studies. Or, if we do get a chance to look through them, we find that we are unable to make any sense of them. What a waste of time! So why bother taking notes in the first place? Well, taking notes is useful because:

- **notes help your understanding of a topic:** you can put ideas down in your own words, or use diagrams;
- **notes help with concentration:** they focus your mind on ideas and concepts;
- **notes help you to link new knowledge with what you already know,** enabling you to see where everything fits;
- **notes help you to keep organised,** helping you to separate important points from supporting detail, assisting with planning and organising assignments;
- **notes can be used to aid revision:** no one has time to read academic books from cover to cover. Notes aid memory.

The important factor in note-taking is learning to be effective in your use of this skill. Equally, note-taking is personal to you: what works for you may not work for your peers. That is why it is usually very difficult to copy notes from a friend: what do all those abbreviations and coloured squiggles mean?

Experiment with your note-taking until you find what works for you. Remember, you may wish to use different note-taking techniques depending on the learning event. One size does not necessarily fit all.

GOLDEN RULES OF NOTE-TAKING

Everybody makes notes in their own way. They can be messily written or colourful and neat, as long as they are fit for purpose, your purpose. If you have a mind that likes to work in lines, you may prefer linear notes. Or if you are a visual learner you may prefer to make your notes using colourful mind maps. Perhaps you prefer words, so making written notes using old fashioned paper and pen, or an electronic device, may be best for you. These note-taking strategies will be explored later in the chapter. Whichever method of note-taking you prefer, the notes should be brief and to the point. The key points should be written down in an organised and structured way.

There is one further point to remember: write notes from lectures in your own words. This will avoid plagiarism when writing your own essays and assignments. Plagiarism is explored in Chapter 7. Also, always write down the name of the lecturer or tutor and the date of the session on your notes, so that if you have any questions you know who to go and see.

TAKING NOTES

Let's start by looking at a range of strategies and skills that will assist your note-taking.

Annotations

If the textbook you are using belongs to you – that is, it is not a library book – there is nothing wrong with highlighting key points and writing comments in the margins or underneath. This is useful if important points can be cross-referenced to other pages in the book. This can save time from making separate, longer notes. If you hope to sell the book after your studies, and you feel nervous about defacing it, then you can always use a pencil, which can be rubbed out later.

Summaries

Summarising your notes is a useful strategy to use while on placement or when revising for exams. Summarising your notes will help you to get to grips with the core points and achieve better understanding of the topic.

Structured Lists

Making structured lists is a useful strategy when used in conjunction with note-taking. It helps with organisation of your studies, identifying tasks that need to be undertaken by certain deadlines. You can also:

- note the key themes in books or during a lecture;
- numbering the key points in a book, perhaps in order of importance;
- identify resources to follow up later.

Keep a Record of Sources

Every piece of information you use in a presentation, assignment or essay needs to be referenced. While note-taking it is useful to record these resources. You may read a gem of a quote in your notes and have no idea where it came from! If this is the case it cannot be used because you do not want to be accused of plagiarism. Noting sources will also assist you in your studies and save you time, as you will be able to obtain an article or book and read around your subject in greater depth, perhaps even referencing it in your own work.

Using Abbreviations

Using abbreviations while making notes saves time. Lots of students use 'text speak', such as Gr8, meaning great, and L8r, for Later. Or, you may prefer to use symbols: see Activity 6.1.

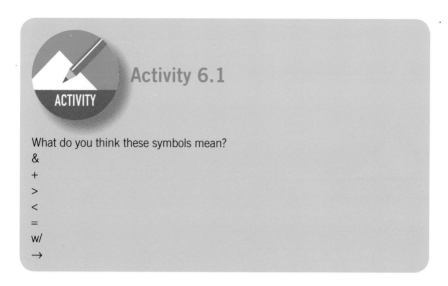

Activity 6.1

What do you think these symbols mean?

&

+

>

<

=

w/

→

If you choose to use abbreviations then you need to know what they mean to you, so it is best to keep a copy of the abbreviations you use while note-taking until they become second nature. Some common abbreviations are listed here:

a/c	account	eds	editor
e.g.	for example	info	information
i.e.	that is	cd	could
etc.	and the rest	wd	would
NB	note this, important	govt	government
		educ	education
p, pp	page, pages	impt	important
para	paragraph	devt	development
ch	chapter	c20	20th century
edn	edition	n/a	not applicable

In health care very few abbreviations are permitted, but unfortunately you may still come across some Latin abbreviations in the field of drug administration. See Activity 6.2.

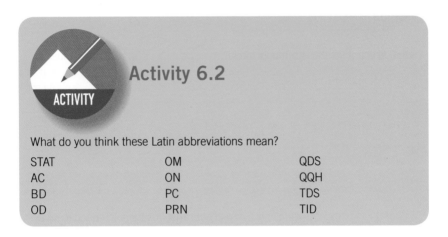

Activity 6.2

ACTIVITY

What do you think these Latin abbreviations mean?

STAT	OM	QDS
AC	ON	QQH
BD	PC	TDS
OD	PRN	TID

Headings and Bullet Points

Headings and bullet points are a useful means of note-taking for those of us who like words. The heading or topic can be written in capital letters, whereas all subheadings can be bullet points. Colour highlighters can be used to separate points. If you want to be really organised, coloured sticky labels can cross-reference similar points in your notes. For example, red sticky labels on sheets in your folder could relate to everything to do with breastfeeding. Anything highlighted in red throughout your notes then also relates to breastfeeding.

NOTE-TAKING DURING LECTURES AND SEMINARS

While listening to lectures or discussions during seminars it is important not to try to record every word that is said, as you will be concentrating more on writing than actively listening to the speaker. It is also important to do some preparatory reading on the lecture topic beforehand so that you find it easier to follow the lecture.

Try out the spider diagram and the linear note-taking methods to see what works best for you. Both of these techniques will be outlined in this chapter. You may need to remind yourself that notes should be brief: only incorporate the main points. Lectures and seminars are verbal environments and you will be given verbal clues to help you to know what is important for you to note down. It is often expected that after a lecture you will expand on the information you have obtained, reading around the topic in more depth. From this you can organise and file your notes under subject headings such as psychology, sociology, communications and clinical skills.

Let me show you a bad example of note-taking: in Activity 6.3 are the notes from one student who attended a psychology lecture. The central theme of the lecture was maternal deprivation. The lecturer posed a question at the start of proceedings: do babies need mothers?

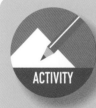

Activity 6.3

Critique the lecture notes below. What do you think is wrong with these notes?

In 1951, BOWLBY produced a report which argued that human infants form a special relationship with their mother, which is entirely different from the relationship which they form with any other kind of person. Bowlby described this process as MONOTROPY (means = tending to become attached to primarily one figure) – which he saw as very similar to imprinting (means = a rapid form of attachment whereby some young animals develop

(continued)

BONDS with its parent or other stimulus). Bowlby considered that the young infant developed a firm attachment to its mother within the first six months of life and that if this attachment or bond was then broken, either by death or by other factors, the infant would suffer serious consequences. He stated that:

...an infant and young child should experience a warm, intimate and continuous relationship with its mother (or permanent mother-figure) in which both find satisfaction and enjoyment. (Bowlby 1951)

Bowlby's study consisted of 44 'juvenile delinquents'. These were adolescents who had been caught stealing and who had come to a child guidance clinic. 17 of these adolescents had been separated from their mothers for a period of time before the age of five years. Comparisons which he made with similar children who were emotionally disturbed, but did not steal, showed that they were less likely to have been separated from their mothers. Therefore Bowlby concluded that MATERNAL DEPRIVATION – being deprived of one's mother during the first 5 years of life – could seriously affect the child's social development, producing juvenile delinquency!

Among his sample, there were two children who were particularly delinquent, and who appeared to have very little in the way of social conscience. This syndrome was described by Bowlby as AFFECTIONLESS PSYCHOPATHY, and he argued that this was an extreme consequence of maternal deprivation.

If the child lacked a special relationship with the mother, it would grow up unable to form relationships with other people. Without relationships with other people, the child would be unlikely to conform to social Norms in the usual way. Therefore, it would fail to develop a social conscience and would become a psychopath, acting out of self-interest without thought for others.

Bowlby produced a list of the kinds of circumstances which were likely to damage children. These were mostly circumstances such as 'war', 'famine', 'death' etc. (he also included 'mother working full time'!!)

Bowlby's thesis concerned the child's need for love, and its provision by the mother: he viewed mother love as absolutely necessary for the normal healthy development of the child and placed great emphasis on the continuity of the mother–child relationship, insisting that adequate love could not be provided by a succession of persons, but must come from one primary source – the child's characteristic monotrophy.

CRITICISM OF THE MATERNAL DEPRIVATION HYPOTHESIS

1 Based on inadequate evidence and on studies with serious methodological flaws, which failed to distinguish the multiple variables involved.

2 Maternal deprivation confuses who the mother is with what she does – a mother may be physically present but not mothering her child and adequate mothering may be provided by someone who is not the natural mother (e.g. fostering, adoption, carer, grandparents).

3 Maternal deprivation fails to distinguish between effects that arise through loss of the mother and effects that arise through a distortion of mothering.

In 1945 a study was conducted of six German–Jewish orphans who were rescued from a concentration camp following the second world war – known as the Bulldog Bank Ophans. During the first year of their life the children were moved from one refuge to another, until they arrived individually in the camp of Tereszin.

Name	Age arrived at Tereszin	Age arrived at Bulldog Bank UK
John	1 year?	3 years, 10 months
Ruth	Several months	3 years, 6 months
Leah	Several months	3 years, 5 months
Paul	1 year	3 years, 5 months
Miriam	6 months	3 years, 2 months
Peter	Under 1 year	3 years

(continued)

At Tereszin they became inmates on a ward for motherless children – they received limited food and medical supervision from inmates of the camp. They had no toys to play with. Two to three years after arrival, the camp was liberated and the children were flown to England. They were observed to be 'wild, restless and noisy'. They destroyed any toys and damaged furniture. They would spit, bite and kick adults. They were observed to care for one another, becoming inconsolable if separated if only for a few moments. It was impossible to treat the children as individuals at the beginning.

These children can be seen to have been deprived of 'mother love'; consequently, their companions of the same age were their real love objects. This case shows that children can survive without their mothers or even mother-substitutes. The orphans eventually adjusted to a new language, customs and began to form emotional relationships with adults. These children were eventually adopted separately. There is no further information on the adult lives of these children. This study did show that some babies can attach to several people, which is at odds with Bowlby's claim.

CONCLUDE

Do babies need mothers? Bowlby's theory, focusing on the biological need on the part of both mother and child to remain close together, stresses a need to bond to one unique female. The majority of research today shows this to be too simplistic and inadequate. The human baby does not bond to its mother with an irreversibility akin to animal imprinting. Babies are flexible and resilient creatures, capable of emotional ties to several adults – and in some cases – to other children.

The human mother is not biologically driven to be with her baby at all times. Many mothers arrange substitute care so that they can go to work etc. There is no scientific evidence that they doom their children to the developmental anomalies predicted by Bowlby.

Children do need physical care and a loving relationship to thrive, which can be provided by someone other than the mother, and not necessarily female – it doesn't even have to be one person – it can be several. Therefore babies need mothering – not necessarily mothers. ADULT MALES CAN PROVE TO BE AS GOOD 'MOTHERS' AS FEMALES (maybe better in some circumstances).

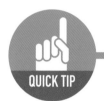

QUICK TIP

Many students use tablets, laptop computers or mobile phones to assist with their note-taking. Some students even use digital recorders to record the lecture as they prefer to 'listen' to the contents rather than keep written notes. It is good manners to ask the lecturer first if you intend record their talk as it may not always be appropriate.

If you are given handouts for a session you will get the most benefit from them by highlighting key words and adding short notes in the margins.

NOTE-TAKING FROM ARTICLES AND BOOKS

You may wish to try making simple written notes while reading information, jotting down key points with headings and subheadings. It is best to find the core of the topic and then make notes around this. Underlining, highlighting and making notes in margins may work well here (see Annotations above). Perhaps you may wish to try out mind-mapping techniques (see below). A good technique to use is something called infographics, which is information presented in a graphic form. This technique gives you lots of information in small bite-sized pieces, making them easy to read and digest. An example of an infographic can be seen in Appendix 4.

SPIDER DIAGRAMS

Spider diagrams are a good means of note-taking for visual learners, keeping the notes brief and to the main point. They are useful also when viewed during revision for exams and for planning essays. There do not have to be themes or links for this type of note-taking; often you can use just one or two words per box or bubble.

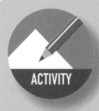

Activity 6.4

Read the text on notifiable diseases. To practice making notes in a visual way, prepare a flow diagram to record the process of informing the authorities about notifiable diseases and a spider graph to record the list of notifiable diseases.

NOTIFIABLE DISEASES

Registered medical practitioners in England and Wales must notify the 'Proper Officer' of the local authority (usually the consultant in communicable disease control, CCDC) of suspected cases of certain infectious diseases. The GP should fill out a notification certificate immediately, without waiting for laboratory confirmation. This form must get to the officer within 3 days. In urgent cases, the GP may need to phone the Officer. These officers inform the Health Protection Agency (HPA) at the Centre for Infections (Cfi) about details of each case of each disease that has been notified.

The notifiable diseases are: anthrax, botulism, brucellosis, cholera, diarrhoea (infectious bloody), diphtheria, encephalitis (acute), food poisoning, haemorrhagic uraemic syndrome, haemorrhagic fever (viral), hepatitis (viral), legionnaires' disease, leprosy, malaria, measles, meningitis, meningococcal septicaemia, mumps, paratyphoid fever, plague, poliomyelitis (acute), rabies, rubella, SARS, scarlet fever, smallpox, streptococcal disease (group A, invasive), tetanus, tuberculosis, typhoid fever, typhus, whooping cough and yellow fever.

Some normally non-notifiable diseases may need notification if there are circumstances which put others at risk; for example, chickenpox in healthcare worker who is in contact with immunosuppressed individuals (known as a public health risk).

Source: Health Protection Agency (2010).

Brucellosis

Bacterial infection that can be caught from animals.

Encephalitis

Condition where the brain tissue becomes inflamed.

Haemolytic uraemic syndrome

Disorder when an infection, usually *E. coli* in the digestive system, produces toxins which cause blood and kidney disease.

SARS

Severe acute respiratory syndrome; a life-threatening form of viral pneumonia.

Streptococcal disease

An infection by a *Streptococcus* species of bacterium (known as a group A).

MIND MAPS

Mind maps may also be known as linear or patterned notes or 'spray diagrams'. This form of note-taking is a useful way of quickly jotting down all your ideas on a subject in a form that contains more in-depth information than a simple spider diagram. Links and themes can be developed from the notes. You start by writing down your central theme and work out with connections through lines that incorporate added information. Mind maps are a useful tool in note-taking when listening to lectures and talks. They can give you a overview of a large topic or subject. Mind maps can also:

- allow you to gather and hold large amounts of information/data;
- enable you to plan routes, to see where you have been and where you are going;
- encourage problem solving;
- be a very efficient method of note-taking;
- facilitate quick reading, musing and remembering;
- allow you to see the whole picture at once and all important details at the same time.

Again, showing a mix of note-taking, look at the information below concerning 'human factors' and see how visual links and mind maps aided my learning:

Implementing Human Factors in Healthcare

The Department of Health (2001) document *Building a Safer NHS for Patients* informed us that although good care is routinely given to NHS patients, an unacceptable number of patients are harmed as a result of their treatment or as a consequence of their admission to hospital. *Why* are these mistakes being made and *where* are they being made? This is where the concept of 'human factors' comes into play, encompassing all aspects of the situation that can influence people and their behaviour. In a work context, human factors are the environmental, organisational and job factors as well as the individual characteristics which influence behaviour at work. It is from these human factors that we can work out why mistakes are being made and patients are being harmed, and then we can plug the holes.

My visual note-taking strategies for the above passage are shown in Figures 6.1 and 6.2.

Once you have got to grips with the key concepts of mind maps, you can develop your own personal style, using colours, images, symbols and upper- or lower-case letters according to importance of the word or phrase. Lines and arrows can be thick or thin according to their importance or the emphasis needed, and will show the associations in your mind map.

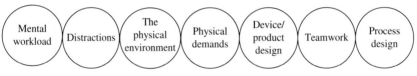

Figure 6.1 Common human factors that can increase risk (data from Carthey and Clarke 2010)

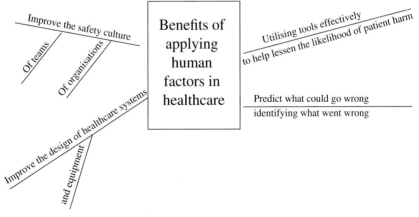

Figure 6.2 The benefits of applying human factors in healthcare (data from Carthey and Clarke 2010)

WHAT TO DO WITH YOUR NOTES

Once you have taken your notes, it is important to keep them safe and work out some sort of system for storing them. You may need to purchase some folders or boxes. Or perhaps you prefer to store your information on a computer, in which case you need to back up your files frequently. Computer hard drives have been known to fail. You may wish to store your notes in folders (on paper or on a computer) using general headings such as psychology, sociology, communications or child development. This is fine as long as you know where to find the information when you need it. If you have made mind maps or written notes during lectures or seminars you might wish to scan them so that they are stored with the rest of your computerised notes. Nothing is more frustrating when retrieving notes for an assignment, for revision or for reference to find that half of them are stored on your computer while the other half are in cardboard folders. Get organised: it will save you time in the long run.

TEST YOUR KNOWLEDGE

From the information below, draw a spider diagram showing what urinalysis detects.

Urine should be straw-coloured. If orangey-yellow it could indicate dehydration and you need to drink more. Cloudiness or an unusual odour may indicate infection. Blood in the urine will make the urine look red or brown.

Urinalysis is also known as a dipstick test. A dipstick is a plastic stick with blocks of chemicals on it and it is dipped into fresh urine to detect abnormalities. The chemical blocks change colour if certain substances are present or if their levels are above normal.

A dipstick test often checks for the following:

acidity: (pH),

protein: large amounts of protein in the urine may indicate a kidney infection,

glucose: any detection of sugar in the urine calls for follow-up testing for diabetes,

ketones: normally the detection of ketones in the urine will require follow-up testing,

bilirubin: bilirubin is a product of red-blood-cell breakdown; if present in the urine it may indicate liver damage or disease,

nitrites and leucocytes: these are a product of white blood cells and if detected may be a sign of a urinary tract infection,

blood: blood in the urine may be a sign of kidney damage or infection, kidney or bladder stones, kidney or bladder cancer or blood disorders, among other conditions.

Vegetarians often have a pH that is above 9.

The preferred sample is an early morning sample (EMU) and one collected mid-stream (MSU).

KEY POINTS

- Golden rules of note-taking
- Note-taking from lectures and seminars
- Note-taking from articles and books
- Spider diagrams
- Mind maps
- What to do with your notes

Bibliography

Branthwaite, A. and Rogers, D. (Eds) (1985) *Children Growing Up.* Open University Press, Milton Keynes.

Carthey, J. and Clarke, J. (2010) *Implementing Human Factors in Healthcare.* How to guide. Patient Safety First, www.patientsafetyfirst.nhs.uk.

Department of Health (2001) *Building a Safer NHS for Patients.* Department of Health, London.

Department of Health (2010) *Health Protection Legislation Guidance.* Department of Health, London.

Hayes, N. (1994) *Foundations of Psychology – An Introductory Text.* Routledge, London.

Health Protection Agency (2010) *Notifications of Infectious Diseases (NOIDS).* Health Protection Agency, London.

NHS Employers (2013) *The New NHS in 2013. What It Means For You.* www.nhsemployers.org.

Sylva, K. and Lunt, I. (1982) *Child Development – A First Course.* Basil Blackwell, Oxford.

Chapter 7

PLAGIARISM AND REFERENCING

Study Skills for Nurses, First Edition. Claire Boyd and contributing author, Beverley Murray
© 2014 John Wiley & Sons, Ltd. Published 2014 by John Wiley & Sons Ltd.

LEARNING OUTCOMES

By the end of this chapter you will have an understanding of how to avoid plagiarism and how to reference correctly.

Plagiarism is using someone else's work, words, ideas or thinking in your own assignment or work and failing to give a reference or credit to that person. In short, it is passing off the work of others as your own, however unintentionally.

Plagiarism, whether accidental or deliberate, can invoke penalties. At the very least you can be given a mark of zero for plagiarism. In the most severe circumstances you may be removed from your course or even prosecuted.

Activity 7.1

ACTIVITY

What acts does the term plagiarism cover? Give four examples.

Copying

Copying could mean submitting someone else's work as your own. This can be from a book, the internet, a fellow student, a previous student or a student from another university. It also includes copying parts of, for example, a book or newspaper article, and not providing a reference.

Failing to Reference Quotes

Quotes are the direct words from a source, be it from a book, journal or website, and includes quotes that a tutor gives you during a lecture. Quotation marks should be used around quoted material in your written work and the source referenced.

Paraphrasing or Synthesising

Paraphrasing or synthesising material from books, journals or the internet includes joining together sentences from a number of sources and not acknowledging them in your writing.

Using Your Own Work

You could plagiarise yourself if you use your own previous work in another assignment and do acknowledging it.

HOW TO AVOID PLAGIARISM

There are strategies to help you avoid plagiarism, which include the following.

- Write all your notes from lectures, seminars and talks in your own words.
- Write down exactly where you read the information or made notes from; write down references as you go along.
- Write down all the books or materials you used for a bibliography.
- Write down and reference any quotes you wish to use.
- If you have a habit of copying then try not to, and put what you read in your own words (but still reference the work).

GLOSSARY

Bibliography

An alphabetical list found at the end of an assignment, arranged by author surname, that lists the sources of information that you have used as background reading. You have not drawn directly from any of this.

Quotation

Using someone else's words directly (needs to be presented in quotation marks).

Reference list

A list of sources that *you have cited* in your assignment. This may be arranged alphabetically by author surname if using the Harvard system of referencing, or numbered if using the Vancouver system.

WHY SHOULD I USE REFERENCES?

In academic writing it is essential to state your sources of information, enabling the reader to check and verify them. Referencing also enables the person marking your essay to:

- see how much research you conducted for the assignment,
- see how much reading you conducted around the subject matter,
- verify the calibre of your sources,
- retrieve any of these sources,
- identify the range of sources that you used: primary or secondary (see Chapter 4).

Marks given for an assignment partly reflect your understanding of the subject matter and marks will be lost if the tutor thinks that you have used too many of your sources' (i.e. someone else's) words and ideas.

WHAT IS SO WRONG WITH PLAGIARISING?

Plagiarism is seen as cheating and is treated very seriously in higher education. Plagiarism can give you an unfair advantage over other students, as academic study is more about the student demonstrating independent learning rather than just repeating other people's ideas and thoughts.

Before you submit your work you will be asked to sign a declaration that the work you have submitted is indeed all your own.

CAN MY LECTURERS RECOGNISE PLAGIARISM IN MY WORK?

Tutors can indeed recognise work that has been plagiarised. There are many techniques, but a few of them are listed below.

- There are computer programs on the market that have been developed specifically to detect plagiarism in written material.
- If the writing style or vocabulary of a student changes, either between assignments or within the same piece of writing, it can indicate that some of the text has been copied from another source.
- A student suddenly getting much higher or lower marks than usual could indicate copying.
- The absence of quotation marks in a student's work can indicate plagarism.

EXAMPLES OF PLAGIARISM

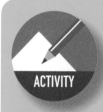

Activity 7.2

Here is a piece of original text on nursing ethics followed by the work of two students who were asked to summarise this text. Is there any plagiarism in either student's summary?

ORIGINAL TEXT

Nursing Ethics

Nursing ethics are a set of principles that concern the nursing profession, sharing many similarities with that of medical ethics:

autonomy	the obligation to respect the personal choices anther person makes,
beneficence	the obligation to do good,
fidelity	the obligation to keep one's word,
justice	the equitable distribution of risks and benefits among people,

non-maleficence   the obligation to do no harm,
veracity   the obligation to tell the truth.

(*Reference*: Breier-Mackie 2006)

Together nursing ethics and medical ethics are known as *biomedical ethics*. However, as nurses focus on care and nursing rather than the cure of illness it has been suggested that ethics of nursing has now shifted more towards the nurse's obligation to respect the human rights of the patient (McHale and Gallagher 2003), resulting in professional dilemmas whereby the nurse cannot focus solely on the medical treatments and ignore the needs of the patient.

The International Council of Nurses (ICN) (2012) states that:

> 'Inherent in nursing is a respect for human rights, including cultural rights, the right to life and choice, to dignity and to be treated with respect. Nursing care is respectful of and unrestricted by considerations of age, colour, creed, culture, disability or illness, gender, sexual orientation, nationality, politics, race or social status.'

The *ICN Code of Ethics* for nurses was first introduced in 1953 and has since been revised and reaffirmed many times since, most recently in 2012. One of the underlying principles of the ICN is that nurses have four fundamental responsibilities:

- to promote health,
- to prevent illness,
- to restore health,
- to alleviate suffering.

STUDENT 1

Nursing Ethics

Biomedical ethics = medical and nursing ethics together:

- **autonomy**
- **beneficence**
- **fidelity**

- **justice**
- **non-maleficence**
- **veracity**

(*Reference*: Breier-Mackie 2006)

Medical and nursing ethics at odds with each other: nursing more about human rights.

The International Council of Nurses (ICN) (2012) states that:

'Inherent in nursing is a respect for human rights, including cultural rights, the right to life and choice, to dignity and to be treated with respect. Nursing care is respectful of and unrestricted by considerations of age, colour, creed, culture, disability or illness, gender, sexual orientation, nationality, politics, race or social status.'

Also that nurses have 4 main responsibilities – to promote health, to prevent illness, to restore health and to alleviate suffering (ICN 2012).

STUDENT 2

Nursing Ethics

Nursing ethics shares many similarities with that of medical ethics:

- autonomy
- beneficence
- fidelity
- justice
- non-maleficence
- veracity

Ethics of nursing has now shifted more towards the nurses obligation to respect the human rights of the patient, resulting in professional dilemmas whereby the nurse cannot focus solely on the medical treatments and ignore the needs of the patient.

Inherent in nursing is a respect for human rights, including cultural rights, the right to life and choice, to dignity and to be treated with respect. Nursing care is respectful of and unrestricted by considerations of age, colour, creed, culture, disability or illness, gender, sexual orientation, nationality, politics, race or social status.

Nurses have four fundamental responsibilities:

- to promote health
- to prevent illness
- to restore health
- to alleviate suffering.

REFERENCING

You should be quite sure which referencing system your university uses: this can be found in your university handbook. Most universities use the Harvard system of referencing, but individual tutors, departments and subjects may determine the style.

Here's a journal article, from the *Nursing Standard*:

Ferguson, L. (2013) Student life - staying the course. *Nursing Standard* 27(29), 64.

When citing an electronic reference, you will need to include the date you looked at it:

Nursing Standard (2013) Students. www.nursing-standard.co.uk/students (accessed 20 June 2013)

Referencing is used to prevent plagiarism. Not acknowledging other people's work is intellectually dishonest and illegal.

When to Provide References

You should provide references whenever you use a source of information for:

- your own inspiration,
- a particular theory,

- specific information, such as statistics,
- a direct quotation.

Where and How to Reference

Using the **Harvard referencing system**, citation in the text of a document should be linked to the corresponding bibliographic reference at the end of the document. In the text you refer to a particular document by using only the author's surname and year of publication. You must also give the page number for all quotes.

If the author's name occurs naturally in a sentence, the year is given in parentheses:

…as defined by Hickson (2013)…

If not, then both name and year are shown in parentheses:

In a recent study (Geddes 2012) in how to increase prevalence of breastfeeding…

If the same author has published more than one cited document in the same year these are distinguished by lower-case letters:

Welsh Government (2012a)
Welsh Government (2012b)

If there are two authors, both their names should be given before the date:

Batalden and Davidoff (2007)

If there are more than three authors, generally only the surname of the first author is given, followed by et al.:

Jones et al. (2013)

Quotations in the Text

There are two main ways of quoting. Either you start with the author (including the date of the publication) and put just the page number after the quote, or you simply put the reference (author, date, page number) after the quote. An example of the first type is:

> Hickson (2013) suggests that '...' (p. 35)...

An example of the second type is:

> The health benefits of consuming probiotic bacteria and yeast (Hickson 2013)...

You will be given a university student handbook explaining the full referencing system to use. You will need to read this information and become conversant with it.

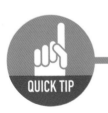

QUICK TIP

Referencing takes a lot of time, noting them all down to use in your assignments. There are many software packages on the market and you may wish to consider purchasing one of these. You can find these packages on the internet using the search term 'reference and citation software' or 'bibliographic software'.

TEST YOUR KNOWLEDGE

1 Give a definition of plagiarism.
2 What is a bibliography?
3 What is a reference list?
4 List the six components of nursing ethics.

KEY POINTS

- Plagiarism
- How to avoid plagiarism
- When to reference
- Referencing

Bibliography

Batalden, P.B. and Davidoff, F. (2007) What is 'quality improvement' and how can it transform healthcare? *Quality and Safety in Health Care* 16(1), 2–3.

Breier-Mackie, S. (2006) Medical ethics and nursing ethics: is there really any difference? *Gastroentererology Nursing* 29(2), 182–183.

Drew, S. and Bingham, R. (2001) *Academic Dishonesty and the Internet: The Student Skills Guide*, 2nd edn. Gower Publishing, Aldershot.

Hickson, M. (2013) Examining the evidence for the use of probiotics in clinical practice. *Nursing Standard* 27(29), 35–41.

International Council of Nurses (2012) *The ICN Code of Ethics for Nurses*. International Council of Nurses, Geneva.

Jones, A., Williams, A. and Carson-Stevens, A. (2013) Integrating quality improvement into pre-registration education. *Nursing Standard* 27(29), 44–48.

McHale, J. and Gallagher, A. (2003) *Nursing and Human Rights*. Butterworth Heinemann, Oxford.

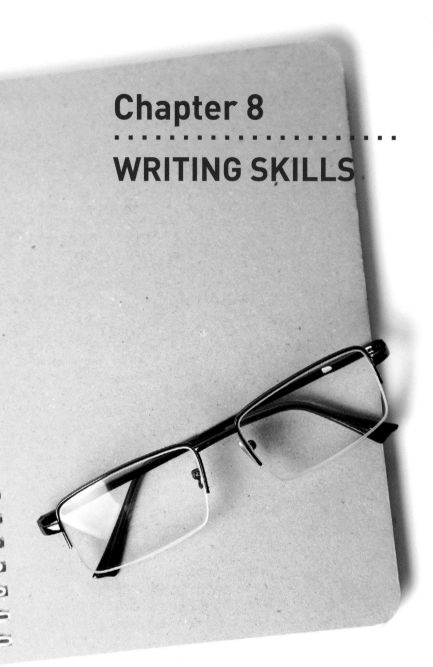

Chapter 8
WRITING SKILLS

Study Skills for Nurses, First Edition. Claire Boyd and contributing author, Beverley Murray
© 2014 John Wiley & Sons, Ltd. Published 2014 by John Wiley & Sons Ltd.

LEARNING OUTCOMES

By the end of this chapter you will have an understanding of how to plan and write academic essays, reports and case studies, of research terminology and of how to present your work.

Assessment at university comes in many different forms, such as essays or assignments, reports, case studies, oral presentations and exams. You will also be asked to research topics and present your findings. In the healthcare setting you will also be required to achieve clinical assessments and get them signed off. You will have a lot to do!

MARKING CRITERIA

The first rule of assignment writing: always look at the marking criteria. The second rule of assignment writing: always look at the marking criteria. Sorry, I got carried away and started to paraphrase the movie *Fight Club*! However, the sentiment still stands: as soon as you get your assignment, look at the marking criteria that your tutor will be using to grade your work. Highlight key words on the assignment brief and make sure you incorporate all the main points asked of you.

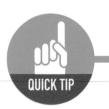

QUICK TIP

During the planning stage of your assignment, tick off the main points from the marking criteria or tutor's feedback form. Make your own checklist according to the criteria that your university uses. An example of one is shown here:

Marks will be allocated for:	Tick when incorporated into assignment
Presentation	
Knowledge	
Comprehension	
Application	
Analysis	
Synthesis	
Evaluation	

THE ESSAY: UNDERSTANDING THE QUESTION

When writing an essay, the first step is to read the question very carefully: it is important to be absolutely clear what is being asked of you. Marks will be lost if you go off on a tangent and deviate from the subject being assessed! It is a good idea to underline key words so that you can keep focused. Remember, the task is to respond to the question asked and it is up to you to select the material you need to answer the question, which must be relevant to the topic.

The essay question will contain key words, such as *define*. In this case you need to give a definition of an aspect of the topic. Other key terms you will come across and need to interpret are shown in Table 8.1.

Table 8.1 Common key words and their meanings

Key word	Meaning
Account for	Explain the cause of
Analyse	Separate into the component parts and show how they interrelate with each other
Annotate	Put notes onto

(continued)

Table 8.1 *(Continued)*

Key word	Meaning
Assess	Estimate the value of; you will need to look at both the positive and negative attributes.
Comment	To make explanatory or critical notes; you may use your own observations.
Compare	Point out the differences and the similarities.
Contrast	Point out the differences only and present the results in an orderly fashion.
Describe	Write down the information in the right order.
Discuss	Present arguments for and against the topic question; you may give your own opinion.
Distinguish	Identify the difference between.
Evaluate	Estimate the value of, looking at both the positive and negative attributes.
Explain	Give reasons; you will need to explain why rather than just define.
Justify	Present a valid argument about why a specific theory or conclusion should be accepted.
Outline	Give the main features or general principles of a subject, omitting minor details and stressing structure.
Relate	Show how ideas or events are linked in sequence; compare or contrast.
Review	Examine the subject critically; to make a survey of
Suggest	Give a range of responses; this question may not have a fixed answer.
Summarise	State the main features of an argument, omitting all that is only partially relevant.
To what extent	Justify the acceptance or validity of an argument, stressing the need to avoid complete acceptance.
Trace	Start with the point or origin of a topic and follow its development or history.

Table 8.2 Interpretations of the question 'Compare and contrast the consequences of blindness and deafness for language development' by degree classification

Degree class	Interpretation
First	Identify the consequences of blindness and deafness for language development. Compare and contrast these consequences, drawing conclusions about the nature of language development. Comment on the adequacy of theories of language development in the light of the conclusions.
Upper second	Identify the consequences of blindness and deafness for language development. Compare and contrast these consequences.
Lower second	List some of the features of blindness and deafness. List some consequences for development including a few for language development.
Third	Write down almost anything you can think of about blindness, deafness, child development and language development. Do not draw any justified conclusions.

Data from Habeshaw et al. (1995).

Habeshaw et al. (1995) showed how students writing an essay on the psychology of child development interpreted the question and gained their degree classifications (Table 8.2).

THE ESSAY: STRUCTURE

Many assignments are written in the form of an essay and will require a title, introduction, main body, conclusion and a reference list/bibliography.

Title

The full assignment question should be written at the top of the page. This is your essay title.

Introduction

The introduction should explain the academic problem as you see it, including the key terms and themes, and should say how you intend to address the question. It tells the reader what to expect and what to look for.

> **Example:** Analyse how a model of learning and reflection can contribute to your own learning and development.
>
> In this essay I will attempt to describe a recent event that happened to me during one of my clinical placements. I will then reflect on how this has been a learning experience for me using Johns' model of reflection (2000) as a framework. I will then reflect on how my own personal beliefs and values may have influenced me during this experience and will further analyse the learning gained through reflection. As part of this reflection framework I will explore whether if I could have done anything differently and if this could have altered the outcome of the event.

The Main Body of the Essay

The main body of the essay should present your case, containing the points you wish to make, with supporting arguments and evidence. It must show the reader that you know your subject. You do this by explaining the subject to the reader in a clear way, using a new paragraph for each new point and by using correct spelling and punctuation, and with no abbreviations. You can use abbreviations and acronyms as long as you write the word(s) in full first with the abbreviation or acronym in parentheses afterwards. Evidence that you use to support or challenge the issues you cover in this section must be referenced appropriately.

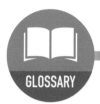

Abbreviation

A shortened version of a word or phrase. Examples include NHS for National Health Service and BP for blood pressure.

Acronym

A word formed from the initial letters of a series of words. For example, laser is in fact an acronym (taken from light amplification by stimulated emission of radiation).

In answering an essay question you may be expected to take one of the following approaches:

- make an argument,
- present an unbiased discussion,
- explain something in a discursive manner.

Throughout the essay, you will be expected to:

- present a balanced argument,
- define clearly the aim of your essay,
- define essential terms,
- use evidence to draw your conclusions,
- use references.

The Conclusion

The conclusion serves two main functions: to summarise and bring together the main areas you have covered in your writing, called looking back, and to make a final comment or judgement. This comment may also include suggestions for improvement and speculation on the future direction of research in the area. The conclusion should not contain any new arguments or ideas. A general rule of thumb is that an assignment of 1500 words or less should not have more than 50–100 words in the conclusion.

USING PARAGRAPHS IN ESSAYS

Essays gain structure by the organisation that you give to the paragraphs. This makes the text manageable and helps the reader to understand it. The beginning of a paragraph should tell the reader what to expect: this is known as the topic sentence. The end of each paragraph should link to the beginning of the next one to keep the essay flowing.

Paragraphs can be linked by phrases such as:

- In spite of this…,
- Although this is true…,
- On the contrary…,
- On the other hand…,
- Another way…,
- Not only…,
- But also…,
- To sum up…,
- You might think that…,
- Firstly…,
- Secondly…,

Each paragraph should not be so long that the reader loses track of the thought being expressed.

PHRASES TO USE IN ESSAY WRITING

There are certain phrases that can be used to serve a variety of purposes in your argument. These are:

- For this reason…,
- To sum up…,
- On the contrary…,
- Equally…,
- In the first place…,
- On the other hand…,
- In spite of this…,
- Therefore…,
- However…,
- By comparison…,
- Furthermore…,
- Alternatively…,
- As a result…,
- In fact…,

Table 8.3 Phrases to be used when starting new sentences

Situation	Phrase
When introducing a similar idea	Also, Besides, Furthermore, In addition
When comparing things	Also, Similarly, But also, Similar to
When introducing an opposite idea	However, Instead, Nonetheless, On the contrary, Whereas, Despite
When introducing an example	For example, Such as, An example of
When emphasising	In fact, Indeed
When introducing an alternative	Otherwise, If
When signalling chronological order	First, First of all, Next, Gradually, Finally
When indicating order of importance	Above all, Most importantly, Primarily, Significantly
When introducing a cause or reason	For, Since, Because of
When introducing an effect or result	Accordingly, As a consequence, Hence, Therefore
When concluding	In conclusion, Indeed, In summary

Data from Severs (2002).

If you find it difficult to think of the correct phrase or word to use when stating a new sentence or paragraph, you may find the table below useful (Table 8.3).

PHRASES TO AVOID IN ESSAY WRITING

- It is a well-known fact... Just because you know something does not make it a well-known fact. Where is your evidence?

- Everyone knows that... Avoid generalisations.

- This is nonsense... Again, where is your evidence? Avoid dismissive, arrogant tones.

USING PLAIN ENGLISH

How often have you needed to read sentences in a document more than once make sense of them? It is not patronising to use simple English when writing, and you can still keep the contents professional. The Plain English Campaign has developed free guides on writing plain English and how to replace words and phrases with something simpler to make the writing easier to understand. See www.plainenglish.co.uk/free-guides.html. Below are just some of the words and phrases that the Plain English Campaign (2001) suggests can be removed from a sentence without changing the meaning or the tone of your writing. In other words, they add nothing to the writing.

- Absolutely
- Abundantly
- Actually
- All things being equal
- As a matter of fact
- At this moment of time
- I would like to take this opportunity
- In view of the fact that
- The fact of the matter is
- To all intents and purposes

From www.plainenglish.co.uk, ©PEC.

ESSAY-WRITING CHECKLIST

When you receive your assignment it is a good idea to work through the checklist in Box 8.1. You can tick each item once completed. But remember, your tutors are there to help you and if you have any difficulties you should contact them. You could show your tutor a working draft, which will assist you in your studies and ensure that you are on the right track. Take advantage of this support.

Box 8.1 Essay-writing checklist

1 Read the question and instructions, analyse and highlight key words and make sure that you understand what the question is asking. If in doubt, ask a tutor.

2 Make a plan and write a rough set of notes outlining the points you are going to make.

3 Generate ideas: make a note of anything which might be relevant to your answer, such as topics, ideas, observations and study materials.

4 Collect evidence/literature, read, make notes and add them to your plan.

5 Complete a first draft with an introduction and conclusion. This may change as you proceed and your ideas develop.

6 Check your work and make alterations.

7 Does the introduction explain the problem as you see it and mention how you intend to handle it? Does it tell the reader what to expect and what to look for?

8 Does the main body of the essay contain the points you want to make with supporting evidence? Is it in a clear format, using paragraphs, correct spelling, punctuation, referencing and abbreviations that have been explained in full first?

9 Does your conclusion summarise and bring together the main areas covered in the writing with a final comment, which may include making suggestions for improvement or speculating on future directions?

10 Does your reference list correspond with the sources you have cited in the text?

11 Go back to the original brief and check that you have answered the question completely.

12 When you think that your assignment is finished, get someone else to check it for you.

13 Make any necessary amendments and submit before the deadline.

Adapted from Hacker (2009).

PLANNING YOUR ACADEMIC ESSAY

When planning your academic essay, you may wish to consider four main points.

1 **Strategy:** you can approach the composition of the essay using a number of different writing strategies.

Some individuals like to start writing straight away and wait to see what develops. Others like to work with small ideas until they perceive a shape emerging. Whichever method you choose, it is a good idea to plan your work. The task of writing is much easier if you create a set of notes which outline the points you are going to make. Using this approach you will create a basic structure on which your ideas can be built.

2   **Planning:** this is the part of the essay-writing process which is best conducted using plenty of scrap paper. Get used to the idea of shaping and re-shaping your ideas before you start writing, editing and rearranging your arguments as you give them more thought. If you prefer, this can be conducted using your computer.

3   **Analyse the question:** make sure you understand what the question is asking. What is it giving you the chance to write about? What is the central issue? Analyse the key terms and any instructions. If you are in any doubt ask your peers, or your tutor, to explain what is required.

4   **Generate ideas:** you need to assemble ideas for the essay. On a sheet of paper make a note of anything that might be relevant to your answer. This might include topics, ideas, observations or other items from your study material. Don't forget to include your seminar and lecture notes when considering what to include. Write down anything you think of at this stage.

REPORT WRITING

You may be asked to produce a report on information you have read or even to conduct your own investigation or study and to write it up. A report is a formal piece of written work that is presented in a different style from an essay. The title of your report assignment may ask the question to be addressed and will indicate your topic. An example title may be: An investigation into the incidents and effects of hospital-induced malnutrition on adult patients undergoing non-minor surgical procedures.

Reports should be written in either the **active voice** or the **passive voice**. The active voice allows you to write short, snappy sentences while the passive is more formal and is generally considered to be more suitable for academic writing. These two voices should not be mixed.

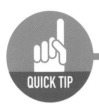

QUICK TIP

The active voice reads:

I recommend …

The passive voice reads:

It is recommended that …

A report usually starts with an abstract, with the next section being the introduction, followed by the main body, conclusion and/or recommendations, and finishes with the reference section. Any appendices are placed at the back of the report.

Abstract

The abstract (Box 8.2) lays out what was done, how it was done and what the main findings showed. It is a short paragraph that summarises the main findings and includes key words/terminology used in the report.

Box 8.2 Here is an abstract from an article in *Nursing Standard* (Haddad 2013) entitled 'Promoting mental health in men'.

Health promotion is essential to improve the health status and quality of life of individuals. Promoting mental health at an individual, community and policy level is central to reducing the incidence of mental health problems, including self-harm and suicide. Men may be particularly vulnerable to mental health problems, in part because they are less likely to seek help from healthcare professionals. Although this article discusses mental health promotion and related strategies in general, the focus is on men's mental health.

Source: Haddad (2013).

Introduction

The introduction of a report should outline the aim of the report and explain why the investigation was undertaken. It usually gives some background to the study topic, and includes a literature review.

Main Body

This may be broken down into subsections such as the study methodology (the form the enquiry took), the results and a discussion of the results. Reports may have a progressive numbering system or be presented in bullet-point form. Each point should be supported by evidence or give examples. If using the numbering system the main sections are given numbers, such as 1, 2, 3 and so on, with subsections being given a decimal number, such as 1.1, 1.2, 1.3, 1.4 etc. The main body includes the discussion.

Conclusion

The conclusion should summarise in a few sentences the main issues arising from the study that can inform nursing practice.

RESEARCH STUDIES

Chapter 5 introduced you to some of the research terminology that you will encounter while critically **reading**; that is, how not to take everything you read at face value. Just as you may be required to **write** a report, you may also be required to conduct a research study of your own and to familiarise yourself with key research terminology. Some examples are given here.

- **Quantitative study:** quantitative research generates numerical data or data that can be converted into numbers. Numerical and statistical forms of analysis can be applied.
- **Qualitative study:** qualitative research is used to explore and understand people's beliefs, experiences, attitudes, behaviour and interactions, generating non-numerical

data; for example, a patient's description of their pain rather than a measure of their pain.

- **Cross-sectional study/survey:** the observation of a defined population at a specific point in time or time interval. Exposure and outcome are determined simultaneously. This type of study contrasts with a longitudinal study, which observes a defined set of people at more than one point in time.
- **Longitudinal study:** a study of the same group of people at more than one point in time. This type of study contrasts with a cross-sectional study, which observes a defined set of people at a single point in time.
- **Epidemiology:** a study looking at the distribution and determinants of health-related states or events in specified populations.
- **Clinical trail:** a research study conducted with patients to test a drug or other intervention to assess its effectiveness and safety. Trial designs may be controlled, randomised, simple (new drug versus old drug) or complex (two or more interventions given independently or together, cross over from one intervention to another).
- **Randomised controlled trial (RCT):** the 'gold standard' for clinical intervention trials. A cohort of patients is randomised into an experimental group and a control group. These groups are followed up for the variables or outcomes of interest. Randomisation reduces the possibility of selection bias in a trial. The test that randomisation has been successful is that different treatment groups have the same characteristics at baseline. For example, there should be the same number of men and women or the same degree of disease severity in each group.
- **Randomisation (or random allocation):** a method analogous to tossing a coin to assign patients to treatment groups (the experimental treatment is assigned if the coin lands heads up and a conventional, control or placebo treatment is given if the coin lands tails up).

- **Quasi-random allocation:** a method of allocating participants to different forms of care that is not truly random. For example, allocation by date of birth.
- **Stratified randomised:** stratified randomisation is used to ensure that equal numbers of participants with a characteristic thought to affect prognosis or response to the intervention will be allocated to each comparison group.
- **P value:** the P value represents the probability of the result of a test of association having occurred by chance if there was no association between the variables. Probability values lie between 0 and 1. If the P value is less than 0.05, it signifies that a result like this could only have appeared by chance 5% of the time if no association actually existed. This is known as statistically significant finding.
- **Variables:** the characteristics that vary between individuals and can be measured or manipulated in the research, such as age and pain levels.
- **Bias:** an unintentional influence or effect which may distort the research findings.
- **Observation:** a data-collection technique that involves the gathering of information through visual means, for example by watching.
- **Reliability:** the extent to which an instrument or technique shows consistency of measurement.
- **Research question:** the specific question that the researcher is seeking to answer through investigation.
- **Triangulation:** where two or more research approaches, data-collection methods or analysis techniques are used in the same study.
- **Sampling:** the technique used to select a portion or part of the population from which the data were collected.
- **Validity:** the extent in which a technique or instrument measured what it intended to measure.
- **Hypothesis:** a statement which is measurable that sets out the expected relationship between two or more variables.

THE RESEARCH PROCESS

When conducting your own research study the framework used is known as the research process. There are eight steps.

Step 1 Identifying problems

Step 2 Searching the literature

Step 3 Critically reading the research

Step 4 Setting the research aims, questions and hypotheses

Step 5 Sampling techniques

Step 6 Data collection

Step 7 Data analysis

Step 8 Interpreting the results

Not all nurses will conduct a research study, but nursing is research-based and so nurses should acquire a knowledge and understanding of research findings. In other words, nurses should learn to analyse and interpret the results of research articles and when reading research reports, to provide the best care for patients. For example, a study may show that a certain ointment is better at treating certain medical conditions than other ointments and change management may occur (changing practice). However, if the manufacturer of the 'better' ointment conducted the study you will need to read the research report in greater depth, looking for any research bias. This is the critical reading covered in Chapter 5. The topic of research is a major topic in its own right.

WRITING CASE STUDIES

In healthcare academia the case study is often used as a learning strategy to apply theory to practice. It can be used to assess a student's

- decision-making skills,
- analytical skills,
- cognitive reasoning skills,
- care skills.

In short, a nursing case study is an in-depth examination of a situation in the healthcare environment that the student has encountered in their daily practice and written about. An example of an introduction to this type of writing is shown.

> The central theme of this assignment will be to explore the individualised nursing care received by a client from clinical placement; it will incorporate a personally planned programme of care using the Roy adaptation model of nursing (RAM). An evaluation of the effectiveness of this care will be discussed prior to concluding.

See Box 8.3.

Box 8.3 The nursing process according to the Roy adaption model:

1. Assessment of behaviour
2. Assessment of stimuli
3. Nursing diagnosis
4. Goal setting
5. Intervention
6. Evaluation

Adapted from: Roy and Andrews (1991).

HOW TO PRESENT YOUR WORK

Presentation of your work is very important, so please do not think that spellnig's not imoprtnat when writign acaedmicaly (that is, that spelling's not important when writing academically). The presentation of your work is the first thing that the examiner will see before looking at the content, and any sloppiness will be reflected in your marks. Spelling, punctuation and grammar *are* important (Box 8.4).

Box 8.4 Punctuation guide

full stop	.	identifies the end of a sentence
semi-colon	;	separates two independent clauses that are not otherwise joined
colon	:	used to separate a statement from an explanation
comma	,	used to break clauses in a sentence or mark items in a list or run of phrases
parenthesis	()	used in place of commas or for referencing
hyphen	-	used to connect compound words, e.g. multi-sensory
dash	–	used in place of parentheses
apostrophe	'	to show possession (the man's hat) or removal of letters (don't forget)

Adapted from Severs (2002).

Remember to check your work before submission. Better still, ask someone else to do this for you. Also, ensure that you have presented your work as required by the university. This information will be in the university handbook: check type size (e.g. 12) and typeface (or 'font'; e.g. Arial, Times New Roman, etc.) and check whether you are required to submit your work with double-line or 1.5-line spacing. Check where on the pages of your assignment your university student number should be placed and where the word count should be shown. You may be required to number the pages of an assignment. As they say, 'the devil is in the detail'. Do not lose marks due to silly errors.

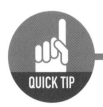

QUICK TIP

Watch out for American versus British spelling in textbooks. Examples include:

American	British
analog	analogue
analyze	analyse
color	colour
diarrhea	diarrhoea

(continued)

American	British
dyspnea	dyspnoea
edema	oedema
etiology	aetiology
fiber	fibre
labeled / -ing	labelled / -ing
maneuver	manoeuvre
millimeter	millimetre
tumor	tumour

GLOSSARY

Dyspnoea

Laboured or difficult breathing.

Oedema

Excessive accumulation of fluid in body tissues.

Prior to submission you will also be required to complete a cover sheet for your assignment. This will show your personal details and include a declaration of authenticity.

HOW TO WRITE A DISSERTATION

A dissertation is usually in the region of 10 000 words and is a piece of writing based on extended reading and some independent research at undergraduate or master's level. In short, it is a demonstration of your intellectual achievement: how you are able to research a topic related to nursing and present your findings appropriately, showing your understanding of key issues and theories, evidence of thought and insight, critical analysis and evaluation. You may choose the subject matter yourself, but remember that this work will take some planning and may take much longer than you first anticipate!

A dissertation needs to be written in the appropriate academic style avoiding colloquialisms and vagueness. Your expressions should be clear and concise with linkage between words and phrases enabling your writing to flow.

A good dissertation will:

- have a clear objective, based on a carefully worked out central question,
- it should be well planned and widely researched,
- include analysis, critical evaluation and discussion; it should not be too descriptive,
- show that you have a good grasp of relevant concepts and is able to apply them to practice,
- be written in an academic style and be structured and expressed appropriately,
- use correct spelling and punctuation, with good use of paragraphs and consistent and correct referencing,
- show your tutors that you have learned how to produce an extended piece of academic work from your training.

A mediocre dissertation will:

- have a general title,
- have a narrow field of research,
- be poorly planned,
- rely too heavily on source material,
- be mostly descriptive,
- contain incorrect grammar and spelling, with little or no referencing,
- be poorly structured,
- not act as your shop window to show your tutors how much you have learned on the course.

How to Produce a Good Dissertation

Spend a good deal of thought on what you would like to write about and consult your tutors to make sure you are on the right track about the topic and expected scope of your dissertation. You will need to focus on specific aspects of your chosen topic, perhaps trying to solve a problem, query currently held beliefs or argue a particular case. It may take weeks to refine your title and agree it with your tutor.

Devise a timetable for your work as a dissertation is a major piece of writing that requires meticulous planning. Remember, your work must be handed in on time unless you have agreed extenuating circumstances with the university. Make an extensive initial reading list, which should be as wide ranging as possible, relevant and with the most up-to-date literature.

If you are going to include a survey or questionnaire, conduct a pilot study beforehand to make sure that there are no mistakes in what you are asking, and that you are asking it in the best way. An example of a poorly written questionnaire question can be seen here.

> How old are you? Please tick an age bracket.
> 20–31
> 31–41
> 43–50

Where do the 31- or 42-year-olds fit in? A silly mistake like this can put your work weeks and months behind.

Your work will require redrafting several times: this is normal. Keep with it. Spellcheck all your work (better still, as previously discussed, get someone else to do this for you). When you have completed the dissertation check the course requirements: does the document need to be bound?

Proposing a Topic

The choice of dissertation topic is likely to be influenced by key factors, such as:

- relevance,
- supervision,
- interest,
- competence,
- scale.

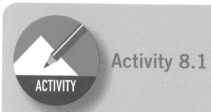

ACTIVITY

Activity 8.1

What do these terms mean in relation to your choice of dissertation topic?

Relevance
Supervision
Interest
Competence
Scale

Structure of a Dissertation

The structure of your dissertation will be according to the university specifications, which you will need to check. As a whole, they do tend to follow the same structure:

- title page,
- abstract,
- acknowledgements,
- table of contents,
- table of figures (if appropriate),
- introduction,
- main body/discussion,
- conclusion/findings,
- bibliography,
- appendices.

You may also be required to include terms of reference, procedure, methodology, an executive summary, a literature review or recommendations, depending on your dissertation.

Referencing your Dissertation

Plagiarism must be avoided, so make sure you have acknowledged all your sources (see Chapter 7). A short bibliography indicates that you conducted very little research, and will result in a poor dissertation, whereas an extensive bibliography indicates a widely researched and academic piece of work.

Knowing When to Stop

Just as it may be difficult to start writing your dissertation, it can also be difficult to know when to draw a line and *stop* writing. You may feel that your dissertation is never going to be good enough and spend hours redrafting and playing around with it. Stop! As long as you have planned well, take yourself away from the work for a day or two and come back to it with fresh eyes and look again at it critically. Make your adjustments, spellcheck it and hand your work in.

TEST YOUR KNOWLEDGE

1   Look through the nursing literature and find two pieces of research, one quantitative and one qualitative. Read these articles and see if you can start to make sense of the research terminology.

2   Look at the essay shown here, produced by a nursing student. It was written some time ago so the contents are very dated and the references old. This branch-specific assignment scored 75% in the Diploma of Higher Education in Nursing Studies. Add paragraphs breaks where you see fit.

An investigation into the incidents and effects of hospital induced malnutrition on adult patients undergoing non-minor surgical procedures.
This assignment will explore the incidence and effects of hospital induced malnutrition (HIM) on adult patients undergoing non-minor surgical procedures, such as an appendicectomy. An argument will be forwarded for the provision of nutrition assessment and continued monitoring (NACM) for surgical patients, with examples of

assessment and monitoring tools in practice. An exploration of the financial cost to the National Health Service of non-assessment and monitoring will be further investigated. However, before proceeding, brief descriptions of the terms 'malnutrition' and 'nutritional assessment' would be deemed necessary. Malnutrition can be defined as an inadequate balance of dietary intake for health maintaining requirements (Oxford, 1991). It is recognised that some patients are malnourished on admission to hospital, however, for the purpose of this assignment, only HIM will be explored. Nutritional assessment can be divided into two sections – an assessment of nutritional status and assessment of nutrient intake i.e. continued monitoring (Reilly, 1996), usually performed by questioning, observation and body mass index (BMI) calculations. Whilst on clinical placement, a thirty-two year old otherwise fit and healthy male was admitted to hospital with suspected appendicitis. After undergoing an appendicectomy, Richard (a pseudonym) made a poor recovery (lethargic etc.). After clinical investigation (serum proteins, anthropometric evaluations), it transpired that Richard was malnourished. It seemed incredible that a patient in 1996, in a modern hospital had experienced HIM – rationale prompting an investigation into the incidence and effects of malnutrition on otherwise healthy surgical patients. Investigations showed that Richard's experience of malnutrition was far from an isolated incidence: Moynihan (1994) states that malnutrition was far from an isolated incidence: Moynihan (1994) states that malnutrition in surgical patients is regarded as a

(continued)

'common problem' with 40–50% of these patients showing signs of malnutrition following surgery, due to the associated trauma of the surgery increasing the need for nutrients, specifically proteins used for the repair of body tissue (Andrewes et al, 1994). Personal experience from clinical practice has shown that nutritional assessment is performed on patients as part of the admission procedure at a very basic level, whereby patients are questioned about their usual appetite and ability to eat and swallow. Patients deemed to be at a high risk of developing malnutrition are then weighed and usually referred to the dietician. However, this basic assessment would appear to be very ineffective due to the high incidence of malnutrition post-operatively (as discussed previously). Andrewes et al (1994) states that an effective nutritional assessment should contain twelve question/factors, such as 'appetite' and 'needs related illness' (Appendix 1). Bacon (1996) further suggests that nurses in the front line should initiate a thorough assessment on all patients, with a multidisciplinary approach with referrals to the Dietician where appropriate. It can therefore be suggested that a nutritional assessment could be incorporated. It can therefore be suggested that a nutritional assessment could be incorporated with the full admission procedures, with minimal increase of time.

Nutritional assessment also involves continued monitoring to assess exactly what the patient has eaten. A good tool for this purpose is the food chart whereby all food consumed is accurately documented, thereby identifying potential problems, such as inadequate intake.

Bacon (1996) states that the food chart is as valuable as a fluid chart and should be completed with the same degree of accuracy. By incorporating this continued monitoring on patients throughout their hospital stay would highlight patients with insufficient dietary intake, such as Richard, whose malnutrition had stemmed from a dislike of the food on offer. Patients otherwise fit and healthy as Richard on admission would not be considered a 'high risk' and may slip through the net becoming malnourished post-operatively. It can therefore be argued that all patients undergoing surgical procedures should be nutritionally assessed pre-operatively with on-going continued monitoring post-operatively with the use of food charts and patient weighing, thereby picking up abnormalities of nutritional status before becoming problematic (Reilly, 1996). The rationale for this NACM on surgical patients is due to the fact that malnutrition among patients in hospital is often not recognised despite the serious clinical (Reilly, 1996, Appendix 2) and financial consequences (Norton, 1996). This is despite the fact that malnutrition prolongs recovery, increases the need for high-dependency nursing, increases the risk of serious complications of illness and increases the incidence of mortality (Davison, 1996). Non-monitoring of nutritional intake could prove to be fatal: Zainal (1995) estimates that in simple starvation, a weight loss of 39–40% can be fatal, but in the critically ill, a much lower weight loss may result in death. Holmes (1991) further states that without lower weight loss may result in

(continued)

death. Holmes (1991) further states that without nutritional support, even in previously 'normal' patients, such losses are accompanied by clinical effects which increase morbidity; nutritional assessment would have the effect of reducing the duration of disability, improving wound healing, lessening the incidence of complications and ultimately reducing mortality. Charalambous (1993) states that during a prolonged hospital stay, malnutrition can often increase or develop for the first time. It is recognised that in-patients stay has been considerably reduced, with emphasis placed on 'care in the community' (as discussed by Alexander et al, 1994). However, it should be noted that patients such as Richard had not eaten for two/three days prior to admission due to pain and nausea, combined with the period of starvation and fluid deprivation prior to anaesthesia (as discussed by Bates, 1994), coupled with the trauma of surgery to bodily systems (Holmes, 1991) all combining to raise the possibility of malnutrition. Indicating, yet again, for the introduction of NACM on all surgical patients, not just those considered 'high risk' on admission. To lower the incidence and identify patients at greater risk of developing HIM post-operatively, calculations of body mass index (BMI) may be initiated on admission, whereby the weight in kilograms is divided by height in metres squared – normal range within the 20–22 region (Davidson, 1996). However, BMI does not give a true reflection of nutritional status (Pennington, 1994); weighing patients on admission followed by daily weights shows more clearly the degree of unintentional or inappropriate weight loss. Reilly (1996) states that the following equation may be used to give a clear indication of nutritional status:

$$\frac{\text{\% Weight}}{\text{loss}} = \frac{\text{Usual weight} - \text{actual weight}}{\text{Usual weight}} \times 100$$

A further method of lowering the incidence of HIM would be to provide diets for individual tastes and preferences. The Patient's Charter (1992) states that:

'You have a choice of dishes, including meals suitable for all dietary needs'.

However, Nazarko (1993) states that food should be appropriate for ethnic dietary needs, describing that some services often assume that the entire U.K. population follow a 'traditional British diet', therefore alienating this group of patients and potentially giving rise to the possibility of HIM – rationale for the training of catering staff and dieticians in special dietary requirements. A thorough assessment of all patients on admission should hi-light special dietary needs/requirements (as discussed previously). It can be further argued that Richard became malnourished due to lack of communication and observation by nursing staff, rationale for the introduction of training programmes by dieticians. Further evidence for the introduction of NACM on surgical patients nutritional needs, and training of health personnel, can be found in the Kings Fund Report (1992, as cited by Harvey, 1993) which states a need to develop the 'recognition of under-nourishment' and to 'increase awareness' of situations in which they occur. This would seem especially important as Norton (1996)

(continued)

states that many Doctors and Nurses do not recognise the importance of monitoring patients nutrition. Nurses are in the unique position of being able to nutritionally assess all patients being admitted as a routine part of the admission procedure, thereby giving more efficient use of resources by involving the dietician for those patients to be in need of nutritional intervention only. The Department of Health (as cited by Holmes, 1994) recommended the assessment of nutritional status becoming routine for all 'older patients', however, it has been shown that vulnerability to malnutrition applies to all surgical patients. Harvey (1993) states that the actual nutritional requirements between young and older individuals varies little between these groups, only the **energy** requirements, further rationale for the introduction of NACM on all patients. Holistic care involves the need for 'individualised nursing' focusing care around the unique needs of the individual (Henderson, 1982, as cited by Reed, 1992). Therefore dismissing sections of society such as the healthy adult on admission, and only performing nutritional assessment and monitoring on the elderly and those considered to be at highest risk could, if malnutrition becomes evident, be viewed as paramount to negligence, further reasoning for the introduction of NACM on all patients. Malnutrition increases the cost of hospitalisation (Holmes, 1996) due to the delayed recovery. Charalambous (1993) states that if 10% of hospital in-patients had their stay reduced by five days as a result of better nutritional support, an estimated £266 million would be saved annually in the U.K. This figure does not incorporate the financial costs to the NHS of patient litigation for negligence. Therefore, it can be suggested, exceeding the cost of implementing nutritional assessment on every surgical patient. Nutritional assessment would appear to be very effective. Queen's Medical Centre perform a full nutritional assessment on every patient admitted to the medical directorate thus lowering the incidence of HIM (Field, 1995).

Routinely assessing every patient nutritionally would give the nurse the ideal opportunity to incorporate Health Education on healthy eating matters (as discussed by Health of the Nation (DOH, 1992), with a view to lowering the incidence of mortality due to unhealthy eating habits by a large proportion of the general public. To conclude, this assignment has argued for the need to reduce the unacceptable levels of HIM by implementing the following factors:

- Nutritional Assessment and continued monitoring (NACM) on all non-minor surgical patients (to include daily weighing).
- Dieticians to raise awareness of special dietary needs, including ethic variations in diet.
- Nurses to be offered on-going training programmes regarding special nutritional needs of surgical patients.
- Nurses to be aware of and recognise the effect of malnourishment on patients and to become actively involved in eliminating the incidence of hospital induced malnutrition.

A multidisciplinary approach is recommended, with the incorporation of Health Education on assessment. It is further suggested to audit the incidence of HIM on for an accurate, up-to-date

(continued)

picture of the cost of this to the NHS. It is hoped that the results of this audit may warrant initiating funding to incorporate the introduction of NACM on all surgical patients i.e. proving to be cost-effective. Moynihan (1994) states that malnutrition in surgical patients is largely avoidable: By incorporating NACM on surgical patients, HIM may be largely eliminated and patients may experience the high quality care to which they are entitled and to which they expect.

KEY POINTS

- The essay
- Using paragraphs
- Using plain English
- Essay-writing checklist
- Planning your academic essay
- Report writing
- How to present your work
- Case studies
- How to write a dissertation

Bibliography

Chandler, D. (2012) *Writing your Dissertation – Some Guidelines for University Students*. Aberystwyth University, Aberystwyth.

Cormack, D. (Ed.) (1991) *The Research Process in Nursing*. Blackwell Scientific, Oxford.

Gould, S. (2007) *How to Write a Dissertation*. Study guides. University of Birmingham, Birmingham.

Habeshaw, T. et al. (1995) *53 Interesting Ways of Helping Students to Study*. Technical and Educational Services, Bristol.

Hacker, K. (2009) *Study Skills Stage 2 – Student Handbook*. North Bristol NHS Trust, Bristol.

Haddad, M. (2013) Promoting mental health in men. *Nursing Standard* 27(30), 48–57.

Johns, C. (2000) *Becoming a Reflective Practitioner: A Reflective and Holistic Approach to Clinical Nursing, Practice Development and Clinical Supervision.* Blackwell Science, Oxford.

Plain English Campaign (2001) *The A to Z of Alternative Words.* www.plainenglish .co.uk/free-guides.html.

Roy, C. and Andrews, H. (1991) *The Roy Adaptation Model – The Definitive Statement.* Appleton and Lange, USA.

Severs, S. (2002) *Study Skills Guide, Disability Support Service.* University of Newcastle, Newcastle.

Swetnam, D. (2000) *Writing your Dissertation.* How to Books, London.

Watson, G. (1987) *Writing a Thesis – a Guide to Long Essays and Dissertations.* Longman, London.

Chapter 9

· ·

ORAL
PRESENTATIONS

Study Skills for Nurses, First Edition. Claire Boyd and contributing author, Beverley Murray
© 2014 John Wiley & Sons, Ltd. Published 2014 by John Wiley & Sons Ltd.

GIVING A PRESENTATION

During your university course, and indeed most higher education courses, you will be expected to give presentations to a group, usually your peers. This presentation may be delivered as a group, or on your own. In health care and academia as a whole, presentations are often used for healthcare professionals to share information with their peers. As a student, you may be asked to prepare a talk on a health-related subject to give to other students. This may take the form of showing how to effectively wash your hands, or you may need to relay information you have read or researched. A discussion usually takes place afterwards to go over the main points.

This may seem daunting, especially if you have never undertaken anything like this before, but learning how to present will stand you in good stead for when you qualify, as many interview panels now ask interviewees to perform a presentation on a topic related to the area they are being interviewed in. For example, presently you are working as a staff nurse in a care of the elderly directorate. A job specialising in pressure area care has come up, for which you are applying. As part of the interview you are asked to conduct a 10-minute presentation on pressure area care.

Whatever the reason for the presentation, it is very important not to go over your allotted time, as you will probably be marked down if you do. If you are on a course it is also important to read the course guidelines for the specifics of the presentation; for example, can you use software such as Microsoft PowerPoint?

Most of us may feel very uncomfortable when standing up to deliver our presentation for the very first time, perhaps in front of peers, but with preparation and practice it may not be as bad as you think. And remember, all your peers have to deliver a talk as well!

BASIC RULES OF PRESENTING: DOS AND DON'TS

- Research your topic well, so that during the post-presentation discussion you will be able to answer questions confidently. Equally, do not try to show off to the group and pitch the talk at too high a level. **Keep it simple.**
- Do not try to pack too much into your presentation: it is a skill to know what to leave in the talk and what to edit out. Remember the time allowed. Very often we try to fit too much into presentations and then have to talk far too quickly, which is hard for the listener. Only present what you can deliver at a reasonable pace. **Don't rush.**
- Interact with your audience, making eye contact, and do not speak too quietly or mumble. Even if you don't feel it, act as if you have all the confidence in the world! **Be confident.**
- Always explain specialist terms to the audience as they may not have yet come across them. For instance, your talk may be on hospital-acquired infections and you mention the NPSA: this will need to be stated in full when you first mention it (National Patient Safety Agency). Consider making handouts for the audience or writing key terms on a board for the audience to see. **Make it clear.**
- Try to relax while giving your talk (see also Chapter 13). Yes, this talk is important, especially if it is to be marked, but the world will not stop spinning just because you 'had a moment' when you became the bunny in the headlights and momentarily froze with fear. It happens to actors all the time. Take a deep breath and try to pick the talk up from where you left off. **Relax.**
- Learn your presentation by heart. Have your script to hand as a safety net, but try not to read from it; instead, connect with your audience. Always finish with a strong closing summary. **Connect with your audience and prepare a strong closing summary.**

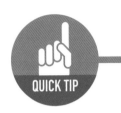

QUICK TIP

Keep it simple
Don't rush
Act confident
Make it clear
Relax
Connect with your audience
Prepare a strong closing summary

PLANNING THE PRESENTATION

To deliver a high-class and well-executed presentation it is essential to prepare. Table 9.1 is a preparation sheet that you may wish to use to help you prepare for a talk. You can photocopy it and fill in your own information.

Table 9.1 Presentation planning sheet

The information I need	Answers
What are the guidelines for making the presentation?	
How long is the presentation and who are my audience?	
What is the title of the presentation, or can I choose one myself?	
What is the date of the presentation?	
Is the presentation to be assessed; if so, what are the marking criteria?	
How long should I spend preparing for my presentation, including research and preparation?	
What visual aids can I use/are there in the room where I will be delivering my talk (e.g. PowerPoint, whiteboard, interactive smartboard, flip chart, posters, etc.)?	
Do I require any handouts?	
What equipment, if any, do I require?	
How will the room be laid out during my talk?	
How long do we have for the post-presentation discussion?	

RESEARCHING YOUR TOPIC

Once you have all the information listed in Table 9.1 you can start gathering information for your talk. Don't go overboard if your talk is only to last 10 minutes. If you go over the time limit you will be marked down and only up to the cut-off time. This may mean that your concluding sentence is not marked. Jot down the main points you want to cover and any extra material you could use if there is time (this may be useful as as padding if you deliver the talk too quickly). When you have made all your notes, separate these into:

- title,
- brief introduction,
- main points,
- summary.

Then you will need to decide how you wish to deliver your presentation.

USING SOFTWARE AND/OR VISUAL-AUDIO AIDS

Using Prompt Cards

When presenting, you may just wish to use prompt cards. This is when you write the main points of the talk on cards and use them as a memory aid. They should only be used as easy-to-read prompts, as eye contact should be maintained with the audience. The cards will keep your talk on track and keep it structured, and will give you confidence in case you 'freeze'. These cards are not for the audience to see.

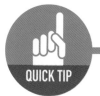

Number your prompt cards and use a treasury tag to keep them in the right order even if you drop them.

QUICK TIP

Figure 9.1 shows some prompt cards for a 10-minute talk on compression stockings.

Card 1	Card 2
• Introduce myself. • I shall be talking about compression stockings. Time: 1 minute	• Why are they used? • Risk factors for DVT. • Other indications for use. • What are they? Time: 4 minutes **Running total: 5 minutes**

Card 3	Card 4
• How do they work? • Styles. • How to put on compression stockings. Time: 4 minutes **Running total: 9 minutes**	• Summary Time: 1 minute **Running total: 10 minutes** Any Questions? (Not usually part of the time allocation)

Figure 9.1 Prompt cards for a 10-minute talk on compression stockings

POWERPOINT

Using Microsoft PowerPoint is a good way of presenting your talk. You may need to get some assistance for this from the IT department at your university or read a manual if you have not used this presentation software before. One of your peers may be willing to help you set up the laptop and projector, so don't be afraid to ask.

As a general rule, on the presentation slides:

- use large text (at least 32 point),
- do not over-crowd the slide,

- use one PowerPoint slide for every 2–3 minutes of the talk,
- do not use flashy sound effects or graphics: they can be very distracting and irritating!

Figure 9.2 shows the same talk on compression stockings, in Microsoft PowerPoint form.

- Slide 1: I would use my first slide to introduce myself and the topic. I mention here that I will be taking questions at the end of the presentation (1 minute).
- Slide 2: first I need to explain the purpose of compression stockings. Then, to cut down on the time factor, I would give a handout to explain the risk factors for DVT and other indications for use for compression stockings (see Box 9.1). The audience need time to read this sheet (2 minutes).
- Slide 3: I explain what compression stockings are (1 minute).
- Slide 4: I explain how they work (1 minute).
- Slide 5: I explain the units of measurement (1 minute).
- Slide 6: I explain how compression stockings are presented: the different styles. I would have examples of the different compression stockings to show (2 minutes). Then I would conclude my presentation by giving a very quick summary and hand out a sheet on how to put on compression stockings (Box 9.2) (2 minutes). Then I can take questions from the audience.

The problem with the above presentation is that I might be tempted to just read each slide word for word. The text on those slides could just be spoken, rather than presented to the audience, and the slides used to relay only the main points, for more impact. If there is any time left at the end of the presentation the process of putting on the stockings can be demonstrated. With visual aids, the stockings and the handouts the presentation can be cut down to just two slides (see Figure 9.3).

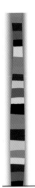

Compression Stockings

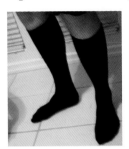

Slide 1

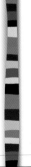

Compression Stockings

- Compression stockings are worn to help to maintain circulation and reduce the risk of blood clots forming in the veins of the legs (known as Deep Vein Thrombosis or DVT). Compression stockings are also called TEDs (Thrombo-embolic deterrent stockings).

Slide 2

What are compression stockings?

- Compression stockings are constructed using elastic fibres or rubber. These fibres help to compress the limb, decreasing the diameter of the vein, and are used to support the venous and lymphatic systems of the leg.

- Beware of latex allergy!

Slide 3

Figure 9.2 Compression stockings, Microsoft PowerPoint presentation

How do they work?

- Compression stockings offer graduated compression with maximum compression achieved at the ankle, decreasing compression as you move up the leg towards the groin. This compression, combined with the muscle pump effect of the calf allows the venous valves, which act as return flow valves, to function effectively, improving the venous blood flow to the heart.

Slide 4

Units of Measure

- Compression stockings are offered in different levels of compression. The unit of measure used to classify the pressure of the stocking is mmHg.

- Compression Stocking may also be classed as Class 1 – Class 3 (which is the tightest).

Slide 5

Styles

- Compression stockings are available in a wide range of colours and sizes. They also come in 3 styles:
  - Knee-High - should sit below the knee
  - Thigh-High - stocking border should rest below the buttocks
  - Waist-High (or pantyhose) – Should rest around the waist with the seams turning vertically up the front of the garment.

Slide 6

Figure 9.2 (continued)

Box 9.1 Compression stockings: risk factors for deep-vein thrombosis (DVT)

- Age over 40
- Being overweight
- Family or personal history of DVT
- Prolonged bed rest (reduced mobility)
- Surgery: especially if lasting for more than 30 minutess
- Surgery involving leg joints or pelvis
- Certain medicines (e.g. contraceptive pill, HRT)
- Pregnancy and childbirth

Other indications for compression stocking use:

- Tired, aching legs
- Varicose veins
- Venous insufficiency
- Oedema (swelling in leg)
- Lymphoedema
- Burn scar

Box 9.2 How to put on compression stockings

1 Insert your hand into the stocking as far as the heel pocket.
2 Turn the stocking inside out.
3 Carefully slip the service user's foot into the sock and ease the stocking over the heel. Check that the heel fits into the heel pocket.
4 Bring the rest of the stocking over the heel up around the ankle and calf; don't pull the stocking. Gently massage the stocking upwards using the palms of your hands.

You can use a fitting aid if required.

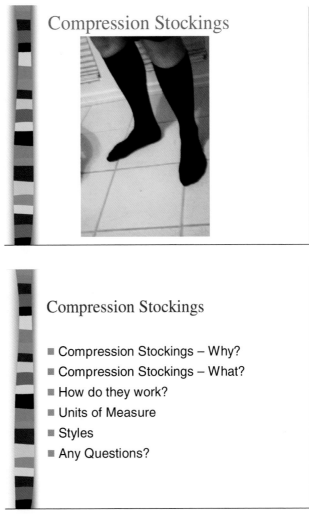

Figure 9.3 Shorter presentation on compression stockings

REHEARSING YOUR TALK

Once your talk has been prepared, you will need to practise, adjusting any slides so that your talk runs smoothly. Have the extra information handy that you gathered while researching your topic, as someone may ask you about the different degrees of compression (Box 9.3).

Box 9.3 Levels of compression used in compression stockings.

Over the counter, stockings may be purchased as:

- 10–15 mmHg
- 15–20 mmHg

Compression stockings may also be obtained on prescription. They are sized by a medical professional such as a district nurse. They come in the following categories:

- 20–30 mmHg
- 30–40 mmHg
- 40–50 mmHg
- 50+ mmHg

Incorrect sizing may cause more harm than good. Always check toes are not restricted.

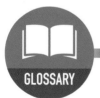
GLOSSARY

mmHg
Millimetres of mercury; unit of pressure.

When you have finished 'tweaking' your presentation have a full rehearsal. Time yourself, speak clearly and do not rush. Microsoft PowerPoint comes with the facility to print a notes page for each slide, but you may be tempted to read from this and not engage with our audience. Keep practising until you feel confident.

KEEPING RELAXED

The more you practise your talk the more relaxed and confident you will feel on the day. Try to remain calm and perhaps go through the Five Senses imagery exercise in Chapter 13. Take deep breaths. You need to be in control. When I am faced with over 100 faces looking up at me at the start of a lecture, I often start with a jokey comment, just to break the ice! But remember, your audience may not find the same things funny as you.

THE DELIVERY

Walk into the room with confidence and set up for your talk, laying out any equipment and visual aids, handouts and turning on computers and projectors. Always prepare well in advance.

It is considered good practice to make sure everyone can hear you at the start of the talk. You may need to project your voice. Keep your voice full and clear. Make sure you can see a clock: you may need to slow down or speed up during your presentation to keep to the time. Don't forget to introduce yourself at the start of your talk.

Look up frequently during your talk and make eye contact with at least two or three individuals each time.

At the end of the talk, sum up the main points; do not just trail off. And lastly, try to smile and relax during your talk and breathe and pause between points.

AREAS FOR IMPROVEMENT

At the end of your talk, and when the dust has settled, consider whether it was a success. Sometimes it is your peers who evaluate your presentation but you can also evaluate your own effectiveness and reflect on areas for improvement. Table 9.2 shows a checklist for you to monitor your own skills. Initially it can show you areas for improvement, and then it can help monitor your progress as your presentation skills develop.

Table 9.2 Presentation self-rating form: rate your effectiveness

Aspect of presentation	Score, 1–5 (5 = effective, 1 = ineffective)
Introduced myself	
Introduced topic	
Smiled at audience	
Made eye contact with audience	
Voice, clear with good projection	
Presentation given at a steady speed (not rushed)	
Used props effectively	
Kept to time	
Summarised points at end of talk	
Answered questions effectively	
Were audience engaged?	
Tutor's comments	

THE POST-PRESENTATION DISCUSSION

During the post-presentation discussion you should respond to any questions as best as you can, being honest if you don't know the answer. Don't just make it up! If you receive any criticism, don't get upset or defensive: take it with good grace and learn from it. Lastly, when answering questions, do not get side-tracked and deviate from the subject: remember to answer the question you were asked. Perhaps finish with the sentence 'does that answer your question?'

GETTING FEEDBACK FROM YOUR TUTOR

Feedback from the tutor is an effective learning aid, showing you areas of weakness (and areas that require improvement) and areas of strength (you're on the right track). Without feedback it is difficult to judge how well you did in your presentation. Perhaps your peers may not be objective with their feedback – 'You were brilliant, darling', 'What a fabulous presentation', 'How do you do it – so confident' – remember, they too have to be assessed by you, so their feedback may not truly reflect your presentation! They want you to be kind to them when their turn comes. They are actually doing you a disservice, as you cannot improve your performance next time and get higher marks. Study your tutor's feedback and aim to include next time anything that received praise and work to improve anything that the tutor says is an area of weakness.

GROUP PRESENTATIONS

During your course you may be asked to give a presentation with a group, instead of on your own. You may prefer this as it does relieve some of the pressure if you feel nervous delivering a presentation on your own. It will also cut down on your workload. However, it does present its own problems. You may be penalised for others making less effort than you, bringing your marks down.

To avoid problems it is important to be well organised and allocate the workload fairly and evenly, and also to establish ground rules from the start. It is also important to keep in touch with your fellow speakers to keep the assignment on track and collate the individual tasks to put together a coherent presentation. You may not necessarily agree on what should be included in your talk and indeed how it is to be presented; remember to listen to your team mates and consider their points. This does not mean, however, that you can't put your own views forward and argue your case.

During group presentation events it is important that everyone makes a contribution and takes a full part in the process. Any problems with the group should be discussed with your personal tutor.

TEST YOUR KNOWLEDGE

Prepare a micro-teach (5 minutes) on how to clean a commode. Hint: Perhaps you would choose to produce a poster for this.

How to clean a commode

Commodes must be cleaned between every single use.

No infection – clean all areas as indicated with detergent wipes.

Infection or Outbreak – clean with Actichlor 1000ppm (1 tablet in 1 litre of cold water)

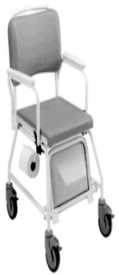

North Bristol **NHS** NHS Trust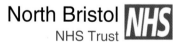

Source: North Bristol NHS Trust and University Hospitals Bristol NHS Foundation Trust.
Reproduced with permission.

KEY POINTS

- Giving a presentation
- Using software/video-audio aids
- Indentifying areas for improvement
- Group presentations

Bibliography

Terry, J. (2012) *Moving On – A Package of Information and Workshop Materials Addressing Skills for Higher Education, to Assist in Building Confidence and Success.* University College Worcester, Worcester; www.worcester.ac.uk/ studyskills.

Chapter 10

. . . .

PREPARING FOR EXAMS

Study Skills for Nurses, First Edition. Claire Boyd and contributing author, Beverley Murray

LEARNING OUTCOMES

By the end of this chapter you will have an understanding of how to study and prepare for examinations, how to answer an exam question and how to write a dissertation.

University degrees are assessed by various methods and this may include written examinations. Examinations are often the cause of much worry and anxiety for students, but with practice and preparation they need not be viewed as a wholly negative experience. They can be seen as a tool to evaluate learning and for self-improvement.

WHY ARE EXAMINATIONS STILL USED IN ACADEMIA?

Examinations are used to establish a student's knowledge base and how effectively this knowledge can be retained and retrieved. At the very least, they can also be used to see how well you work under pressure! They are not solely a test on how much information you can remember and recount from your lectures or textbooks; they are also about how you *use* this knowledge.

STUDYING AND PREPARING FOR EXAMS: TIPS FROM PAST STUDENTS

* Firstly, you will need to get organised: plan your revision timetable. Spread this out over a long period of time to avoid last-minute cramming. University study is more about communicating an understanding of a subject rather than just memorising information. When you plan your revision timetable you will need to be realistic. Most people cannot sustain studying for large chunks of time, so give yourself plenty of breaks and remember to plan some recreation time.

- You will have worked out by now what sort of learner you are (Chapter 2). Prepare your workspace accordingly. Visual learners may make mind maps and enjoy music playing in the background to achieve optimum study.
- To study efficiently you will need to be rested and relaxed. Too many all-night parties will not help your revision as you will be constantly tired, unless of course you are a lucky individual who requires less sleep than most.
- Eat well and keep healthy, drinking plenty of water. To sit exams you need to be in tip-top health. Tea and coffee and stimulant drinks will give you temporary boosts of energy but will not help your concentration levels: water is best for hydration.
- Time your revision. It may not be best after you have just worked a very busy shift and feel exhausted.
- Organise a revision group: they can help with gaps in your knowledge, and you can help others too. This need not be conducted in person, and can be undertaken on the internet.
- Don't avoid study topics just because they are hard for you: you will probably need to spend more time on these areas.
- If you can, get hold of some past exam papers. You will gain confidence if you see what format a paper takes. Write timed answers from these past papers.
- Don't just read your lecture notes and seminar notes over and over again: make more sense of them by linking the topics.
- Keep testing yourself, reciting main issues in the exam topic.
- Double check exam dates, times and venues. Make sure you have all the equipment you require for the exam the night before. Some examinations allow the student to take books in with them.
- Find out what type of exam you are taking, whether essay-type questions, multiple choice, short answers, open-books or seen exam.

MEMORY STRATEGIES

Students often find strategies to help them remember important facts and/or points. This may take the form of simply making sense of the learning, then putting the information into your own words. Some people like to make the information more memorable by making sounds or images to go with the information to form mental pictures and stories to go with the ideas. Some like to draw infomatic posters to study every time they pass to help retain the information. Mnemonics are also a useful revision tool to assist when facts need to be learned. This is where the first letter of each word is used to create an easily remembered phrase or word. Below is an example of a mneumonic for remembering the layers of the skin's epidermis.

Corny Lucy's Granny Spins Germs

Stratum **corn**eum
Stratum **luci**dum
Stratum **gran**ulosum
Stratum **spin**osum
Stratum **germ**inativum

Find out what works for you.

THE NIGHT BEFORE THE EXAMINATION

The night before the exam, keep calm. Go to bed at a reasonable time, leaving a good gap between your last-minute revision and sleeping. If you study too late your head will be buzzing with information and you won't get enough sleep. Try to relax with friends or play some music, watch television, read a book or take a relaxing bath or shower: chill.

ANSWERING EXAMINATION QUESTIONS

Once in the exam room, read the instructions carefully. You will need to:

- work out your timings (if you are required to answer four exam questions, each attracting 25% of the marks, then divide your timings into quarters);
- read the questions carefully (read through the test paper quickly, just to see what you are dealing with, and then re-read it slowly);
- if you are not required to answer all the questions on the exam paper then choose the questions that you can answer the best (make a note of these questions and plan your answers);
- decide on your question order (some people like to answer their best question first to give them confidence; others like to start with their weakest question first);
- before the end of the examination check that you have actually answered each question fully.

WHAT TO DO IF YOUR MIND GOES BLANK

This is the biggest fear for most students, but don't panic. Put your pen down. Close your eyes. Sit back for a moment and relax. Take some deep breaths. Then go back to the examination, leave a gap and carry on and go back to this point later when the creative juices start to flow again (not your tears!).

WHAT TO DO IF TIME IS RUNNING OUT

Again, don't panic. If you have mis-timed your answers, divide up your remaining time to cover the questions you need to answer, even if this just consists of bullet points with a point or two as support. At least you will pick up a few marks.

EXAMS COME IN MANY DIFFERENT SHAPES AND SIZES!

Exams may not always ask you to impart your knowledge in writing. They may also ask you to show your knowledge by labelling or drawing anatomy diagrams.

Activity 10.1

ACTIVITY

Can you label the diagram below? (Figure 10.1)

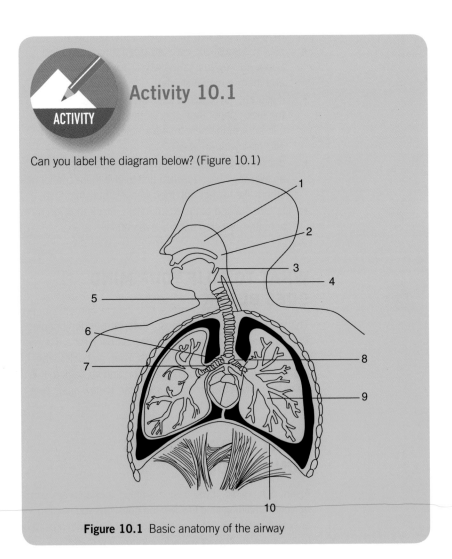

Figure 10.1 Basic anatomy of the airway

ASSESSMENTS

You may also be assessed on your competency in performing a clinical skill. This type of observed assessment, which can be conducted at university in a clinical skills laboratory or classroom, or on clinical placement, is designed to show that you have the knowledge and skills for safe and effective practice when working without direct supervision. Some of the skills in a practical assessment will include cannulation and venepuncture. There are many assessment criteria for competency assessment, one of which is the Fearon scale (Table 10.1). According to Fearon (1998), who adapted this

Table 10.1 Rating scale: levels of achievement

Level	Associated statement
0	Cannot perform the activity satisfactorily to participate in the clinical environment
1	Can perform the activity *but* not without constant supervision and some assistance
2	Can perform the activity satisfactorily but requires some supervision and/or assistance
3	Can perform the activity without supervision and/or assistance
4	Can perform the activity satisfactorily without assistance and/or supervision with more than acceptable speed and quality of work
5	Can perform the activity satisfactorily with more than acceptable speed and quality of work, and with initiative and adaptability to special problem situations
6	Can perform the activity with more than acceptable speed and quality, with initiative and adaptability, and can lead others in performing the activity

Reference: Fearon (1998).

rating scale for nursing, *competence is achieved at level 3.* It is only in more advanced practitioners that you would expect to see higher levels, 4 and above, as the practitioner moves towards achieving expertise in the technique.

Whichever clinical competency rating scale is used, the scale should have three functions for the assessment to be robust:

- to evaluate clinical behaviours,
- to provide a predetermined range of reference,
- to provide a label for each reference/scale point.

TEST YOUR KNOWLEDGE

Conduct a literature search on natural rubber latex to answer this examination question.

> What is a natural rubber latex allergy and what is its relevance in healthcare? (500 words)

KEY POINTS

- How to study and prepare for exams
- Memory strategies
- The night before the exam
- Answering exam questions
- Assessments

Bibliography

Fearon, M. (1998) Assessment and measurement of competence in practice. *Nursing Standard* 12(22), 43–47.

University of Albany (nd) Expert tips to prepare for exams. www.albany.edu/main/features/2004/12-04/1exams/exams.html.

Chapter 11

WRITING A PORTFOLIO

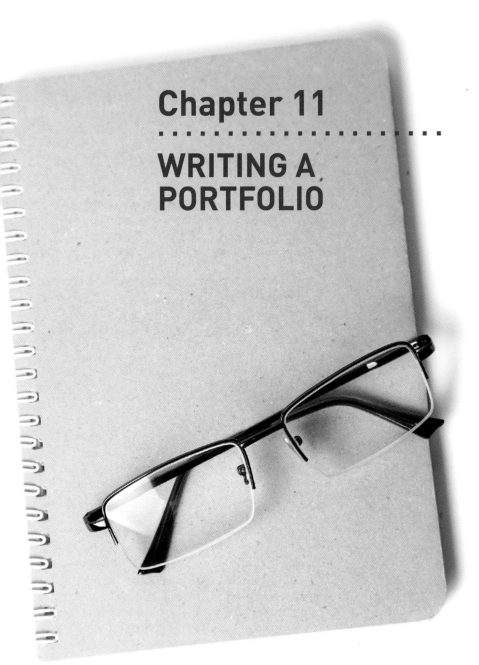

Study Skills for Nurses, First Edition. Claire Boyd and contributing author, Beverley Murray
© 2014 John Wiley & Sons, Ltd. Published 2014 by John Wiley & Sons Ltd.

LEARNING OUTCOMES

By the end of this chapter you will have an understanding of how to create and maintain a professional portfolio.

WHAT IS A NURSING PORTFOLIO?

A nursing portfolio is a record of your professional development, a folder containing your personal and professional goals, growth and achievements. It is also the place to store your certificates, competency paperwork and record of study days. It is most certainly not a glorified curriculum vitae (CV).

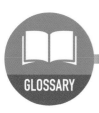

GLOSSARY

Portfolio

A collection of evidence, usually in written form, of both the products and processes of learning. It attests to achievements and personal and professional development, by providing critical analysis of its contents (McMullan et al. 2003).

All students should start a portfolio at the beginning of their course, and tutors will assist with this. At the end of your training, when you start going for job interviews, it can be produced to showcase what you have learned during your training, what you perceived as your strong points and areas you wish to improve. Then, once you have qualified, your portfolio can be transferred seamlessly from being a student portfolio to become a qualified nursing or midwifery professional portfolio. All nurses and midwives are required to keep a portfolio as part of their PREP (that's Post-Registration Education and Practice) requirements to provide a high standard of practice and care. The portfolio can be used as evidence that you have indeed fulfilled these requirements in order to remain on the Nursing and Midwifery Council (NMC) register.

Once a portfolio has been started it should be kept up to date, with information added as you attend study days, and older information removed. The portfolio is your property and should therefore be designed to suit your needs. Portfolios can be kept electronically, but many employers will want to see a hard copy at your interview so that they can look through, view your certificates and thank-you cards, etc., from placements. Of course, these can also be scanned for electronic storage. A portfolio is also good place to store all your certificates, keeping them together.

PREPARING YOUR PORTFOLIO

You can purchase specialised nursing portfolios, but it is just as good to make your own, selecting a good four-ringed binder. As the portfolio is a professional tool, so a plain, coloured binder should be selected. Folders with comic characters or pictures of cannabis plants on (both of which I have seen) do not show your fun side, as one student told me they did, any more than an email account beginning drunkanbum@.... Neither are professional and they should never be used in a professional capacity.

Next you will need some plastic wallets to place your certificates and other precious paper records in (certificates should not have holes punched and be placed directly in the folder). You also need some dividers to divide the portfolio into sections.

You will need to start collecting together your certificates, record of study days, assessment-of-practice records, reflections and anything else you will be adding to your portfolio.

NMC REQUIREMENTS

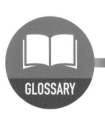

GLOSSARY

CPD
Continuing Professional Development

NoP
Notification of Practice

PREP
Post-Registration Education and Practice

As a qualified nurse or midwife you will adhere to the Nursing and Midwifery Council's (2008) code of conduct. The NMC maintains a register of all nurses and midwives who have fulfilled the Council's registration requirements and are therefore able to practice in the UK and the Islands. This register safeguards the health and well-being of the public.

When you are qualified you will pay an annual registration fee and will need to sign a Notification of Practice (NoP) form. This form asks you to declare that you have met your PREP requirements and are of good health and good character. There are two PREP standards, as follows.

1 **PREP Practice Standard:** You must have worked in some capacity of your nursing or midwifery qualification during the previous 3 years for a minimum of 450 hours, or undertaken an approved return to practice course (for nurses who have let their registrations lapse).

2 **PREP Continuing Professional Development (CPD) Standard:** You must have undertaken at least 35 hours of learning activity relevant to your practice and recorded your CPD over the 3 years prior to the renewal of your registration.

So you can see that your portfolio is not just a nice thing to have, but a professional requirement. Once you are qualified and on the NMC register the NMC can ask to see evidence of your CPD any time it wishes. Failure to comply with CPD can mean removal from the register and loss of your right continue a career as a registered nurse or midwife. You can view the full NMC *Code of Conduct* and *PREP Handbook* on the Council's website (www.nmc-uk.org; see also the Bibliography at the end of this chapter).

SETTING OUT YOUR NURSING PORTFOLIO

The portfolio should include a number of core components, but can be laid out any way you wish. Box 11.1 shows how I laid out my professional nursing portfolio.

Box 11.1 Layout for a professional nursing portfolio

Title page

Contents page

Section 1: Biographical information: name, address, contact details, nursing and midwifery PIN number and date of renewal.

Section 2: Educational background, including further education, higher education (e.g. Diploma in Counselling), registered qualification (e.g. nursing qualification, Certificate in Education) and professional diplomas/certificates (e.g. City and Guilds courses in massage, aromatherapy, etc.); institution names and dates should be given.

Section 3: This is the section in which I have placed all my professional certificates.

Section 4: Employment history, starting with the most recent first. Here I have given an overview of the job in question and my duties. For my present position I have added my job description. This is also the section where I have added my CV, which includes a small section on my interests and hobbies and my reference contacts. A CV should not be more than one piece of A4 paper, covering two sides.

Section 5: Continuing professional development (CPD): this is where I have placed my records of study days (e.g. intravenous study day, venepuncture, cannulation, male urinary catheterisation, tracheostomy study day). I have also added the dates I attended updates of these sessions, with a small written piece about what I have learned during these training sessions. It is in this section that I have recorded my hours spent studying. This section also contains the titles and dates of mandatory training events attended, and when I am required to re-attend these events (e.g. 2- or 3-yearly). In this section I have also written brief pieces about conferences and lectures that i have attended, and also articles I have read that may have made a difference to my nursing practice.

Section 6: This is the section where I insert my annual appraisal paperwork and my personal and professional goals for the short and long term; my action plans.

Section 7: Here I add my reflective pieces that enhance my practice. I also add my SWOT analysis (see below), identifying my strengths and weaknesses.

Section 8: This is where I have inserted professional articles that I have had published, or details of talks I have given or presentations I have delivered.

Section 9: This is where I document my participation in committees, or extra responsibilities I have taken on.

Section 10: This is where I identify any awards I have received, or been put forward for, and also where I put letters or thank-you cards from patients, their families or my peers. (Remember to remove any identifying details on such items, for confidentiality purposes.)

As a student, your portfolio can be adapted in Section 4 to include copies of university competencies that you have had signed off, your preceptor's grading/remarks on your placements and, as you progress through your training, study days attended while on placement. Don't forget to include 'bedside teaching sessions' by peers. Section 6 can include agreed targets that you have discussed with your personal tutor. Section 7 can include assignments for which received high marks, and also case studies. Just be inventive. Your portfolio is not meant to be static, but forever evolving.

KEEP IT BRIEF

One point to note: although it seems that a lot of information goes into a portfolio you will need to edit it quite heavily. I once saw a qualified nurse bring two great, heavy portfolio folders to a job interview. They seemed to contain her whole life story, with every single course she had attended since qualification. Make sure that your portfolio is light enough to pick up easily and that it only contains information that is relevant to now.

Your portfolio should look professional and the written text in it should contain no spelling mistakes, so always

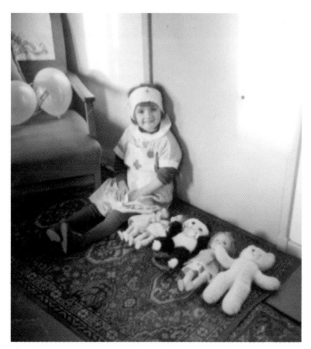

Figure 11.1 I always wanted to be a nurse

spellcheck your work. There is an opportunity for you to add anything that you think will enhance the portfolio. For instance, I added a time line to Section 6 of my portfolio, starting with a photograph of me aged 4 alongside a caption stating that I had always wanted to be a nurse (Figure 11.1). The time line continued to the present day, and had my long-term and short-term goals laid out. Make the portfolio personal to you. There is absolutely no need to include a photograph of yourself on a drunken night out with your colleagues to show what a good team worker you are! That would not be professional.

STUDENT PORTFOLIOS

As a student nurse you will be working long hours, writing assignments and attending university, but you should not see your portfolio as 'just another thing they want us to do'.

The portfolio is an active learning tool and will actually help you with your course. It is your resource. It will:

- show how your knowledge and skills have developed during the course on an individual and a professional level;
- provide evidence of personal and professional achievements;
- demonstrate how you link theory to practice (and vice versa);
- show your personal and professional goals;
- demonstrate the practical application of underpinning knowledge;
- demonstrate the practical ability you have achieved during your course;
- show how you have developed your key skills, such as by reflective practice.

REFLECTIVE PRACTICE

Reflective practice is a process which enables you to achieve a better understanding of yourself, your skills, competencies, knowledge and professional practice. Although most of us engage in thinking about experiences before, during or after an event, we need to document the experience to identify clearly what we have *learned* from the experience. Writing this down gives you the opportunity to comment on your own actions and experiences. It will help you explore how your actions could or should impact on your professional development by looking at what you did right, and how you could have made the situation better. You may have had a bad day on a placement and can use reflection to improve future experiences. Reflection will help you to plan for the future and to implement improvements in your own performance.

There are many reflection tools that you can use, one of which is the Gibbs reflective cycle (Gibbs 1988). You can make up your own along the lines of the list in Box 11.2, but the reflective process always should include a description, an account of how you felt, an evaluation, an analysis, a conclusion and an action plan.

Box 11.2 List of points for reflection

1   What happened? Describe the incident.
2   What did you think/feel?
3   Your evaluation of the experience: what went well?
4   Your analysis of the situation: what could have gone better?
5   Conclusion: what else could you have done? What have you learned from this experience?
6   Action plan: if the situation arose again, what would you do differently?

Adapted from Gibbs (1988).

Activity 11.1

Using the template in Box 11.2, write a reflective piece on something that has happened to you while on placement: it can be something good or something not so good.

REFLECTION IN ACTION

Reflective pieces should go into your portfolio and will show evidence of you learning in action. When I was newly qualified I unintentionally upset a very experienced nurse and used reflection to make sense of the whole situation. The staff nurse was using intravenous (IV) fluid bags as heel protectors on immobile patients (part 1 of the reflection process; see Box 11.2). I spoke to her, stating that fluid bags were not the correct equipment to prevent pressure sores on patient's heels and was told that I did not know what I was talking about and this was practice that had been going on for years. I felt very belittled (part 2 of the reflection process).

I immediately gathered up all the research I could find, showing that this practice was actually doing more harm than good in pressure area care (part 3 of the reflection process). I informed the ward manager of my findings and spoke to the tissue viability nurse, who was horrified at this practice.

The nurse was spoken to and agreed to change her practice. I dreaded working with the nurse, who subsequently made my life difficult, accusing me of 'stabbing her in the back' (which of course I had not done). When I analysed the situation (part 4 of the reflection process) I realised that the nurse was very hurt by my actions, but I had discussed this with her at the start and she had been unwilling to embrace up-to-date practice and was causing harm to the patients. But perhaps I could have taken the research findings to the nurse before going to the manager and reporting her for bad practice (part 5 of the reflection process). My action plan (part 6 of the reflection process) stated that I would go to the tissue viability nurse, who could enforce correct practice. I would not let bad practice go unchecked because I am the patient's advocate, but I should be much more sensitive in my approach.

My current portfolio contains four pieces of reflection, with the above example having long been replaced. Material in a portfolio should be updated annually or bi-annually.

SWOT

SWOT stands for strengths, weaknesses, opportunities and threats. SWOT analysis is a type of self assessment that is very common in the healthcare work environment and it is usually included in a portfolio. Your own self knowledge, other people's perception of your skills and abilities and an understanding of the context in which you work will help you analyse the personal and organisational factors relevant to your development. A periodic SWOT analysis is useful to focus your activities.

Figure 11.2 shows a SWOT analysis. As an example, a strength could be that you are a good team worker, and

Strengths	Weaknesses
What do I do really well?	What could I do better?
Opportunities	**Threats**
What opportunities.exist or may become available to help me to achieve my goals?	What barriers are there? What/who may inhibit my progress?

Figure 11.2 SWOT analysis

a weakness may be that your time management is poor. In this case you could speak to your tutor or preceptor to help you improve your time-management skills. It may be a worry that as you gain experience in your clinical placement your increased workload will put further time pressues on you. being aware of this and working to improve this weakness will help you avoid any problems as your responsibilities increase.

TEST YOUR KNOWLEDGE

1 Complete a SWOT analysis of your first week in clinical practice and put it in your portfolio.
2 Place the reflective piece you wrote for Activity 11.1 into your portfolio.

KEY POINTS

- Writing a nursing portfolio
- Reflective practice
- SWOT analysis

Bibliography

Evans, M. (2004) Listen up. Keeping a portfolio has boosted my confidence in my own abilities. *Nursing Times* 100(43), 18.

Gibbs, G. (1988) *Learning by Doing: A Guide to Teaching and Learning Methods.* Oxford Centre for Staff and Learning Development, Oxford Polytechnic. Further Education Unit, London.

Hull, C., Redfern, L. and Shuttleworth, A. (2005) *Profiles and Portfolios. A Guide for Health and Social Care*, 2nd edn. Palgrave MacMillan, Basingstoke.

McMullan, M., Endacott, R., Gray, M.A., Jasper, M., Miller, C.M.L., Scholes, J. and Webb, C. (2003) Portfolios and assessment of competence: a review of the literature. *Journal of Advanced Nursing* 41(3), 283–294.

Nursing and Midwifery Council (2008) *The Code: Standards of Conduct, Performance and Ethics for Nurses and Midwives.* NMC, London; www.nmc-uk.org/code.

Nursing and Midwifery Council (2011) *The PREP Handbook.* NMC, London; www.nmc-uk.org.

Oermann, M. (2002) Developing a professional portfolio in nursing. *Orthopedic Nursing* 21(2), 73–82.

Chapter 12
. . . .
LEARNING IN PRACTICE

Study Skills for Nurses, First Edition. Claire Boyd and contributing author, Beverley Murray
© 2014 John Wiley & Sons, Ltd. Published 2014 by John Wiley & Sons Ltd.

LEARNING OUTCOMES

By the end of this chapter you will have an understanding of the meaning of bedside teaching, or learning in practice, as a teaching strategy.

The Nursing and Midwifery Council (NMC) requires nursing and midwifery students to complete 50% of their training in the clinical area (Nursing and Midwifery Council 2008). In a clinical placement students are supervised by qualified health professionals and their mentors. It is the mentor's role to support the student and to sign off assessed skills against required competencies in documentation from the university. Part of a mentor's role is to provide (or facilitate) bedside teaching events, as teaching does not occur only in the formal classroom setting.

BEDSIDE TEACHING: WHAT IS IT?

Teaching at the bedside is defined as teaching in the presence of a patient. However, it is far wider than this, as not all clinical placements occur in the acute hospital setting. They can also be in a long-term care setting, a clinic, the patient's home and many other places. It is therefore more appropriate to state that bedside teaching refers to patient-based and patient-orientated teaching and learning. It should be remembered that maternity students do not refer to the expectant mother or newborn baby as 'patients' as such, and so it may be more appropriate to refer to this type of learning opportunity as **learning in practice**.

NOTE: teaching sessions for learning in practice must always include the patient, client or service user.

WHAT ARE THE BENEFITS OF LEARNING IN PRACTICE?

Learning in Practice brings with it unique benefits to the student's learning.

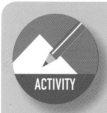

Activity 12.1

List six potential benefits of learning in practice for the student nurse.

EFFECTIVE LEARNING IN PRACTICE TEACHING

Healthcare professionals have traditionally learned their skills in an apprenticeship-type model whereby novices observe their experienced colleagues at work, and pick up these skills.

> Observation > Understanding > Practice
> *Source*: Gill (2007).

If these logical steps are not adhered to, this model of learning runs the risk of:

- being haphazard,
- not adequately covering the content of the curriculum,
- leading to novices being asked to perform tasks for which they may be unprepared and unsupervised,
- encouraging the development of poor skills as well as good ones,
- leaving the learner feeling generally overwhelmed by the need to make sense of what they are learning.

Adapted from Gill (2007).

THE EFFECTIVE TEACHER

In whatever healthcare environment that you, the student nurse, has been placed, teaching can occur in most areas.

Learning in practice should have key traits. The effective clinical teacher should:

- encourage active participation rather than passive observation and demonstrate *positive attitudes* towards teaching;
- spend time with the learner to establish previous knowledge base and negotiating what will be taught and what you may wish or need to learn.

EXAMPLE: INTRAVENOUS FLUIDS

Here is an example of mentor–student learning in a practice teaching session about intravenous (IV) fluids. A student nurse on her first placement has never seen a bag of IV fluids being set up ready for administration to the patient (Figure 12.1). The mentor has thought about the learning objectives of this teaching session and related them to the

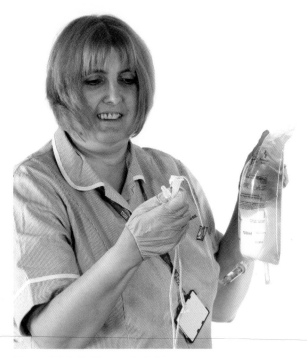

Figure 12.1 Setting up IV fluids

student, which were that by the end of the session the student will be able to:

- identify the correct patient and obtain informed consent,
- demonstrate an awareness of the potential risk factors and how to prevent complications,
- identify the correct prescribed fluid,
- identify the correct drip rates, total volume and duration of infusion,
- appreciate the importance of asepsis and maintain aseptic technique throughout the procedure,
- demonstrate reasonable safe practice.

The teaching is run as a question and answer session, as follows.

> Mentor: Why do we give IV fluids to patients?
>
> Student nurse: To hydrate the patient if they are dehydrated.
>
> Mentor: Yes, can you think of any more reasons why we would administer IV fluids?
>
> Student nurse: Not sure, does a blood transfusion count?
>
> Mentor: Yes, due to hypovolaemic shock, a massive blood loss. The main reasons for administering IV fluids are patient is nil by mouth (i.e. they have no swallow reflex, pre-surgery or after trauma), dehydration, hypovolaemic shock, electrolyte replacement and administration of drug therapy.
>
> Mentor: Can you name any of the types of IV fluid?
>
> Student nurse: No.
>
> Mentor: Well, they can be crystalloids, such as normal saline 0.9% or 5% dextrose, colloids such as gelofusine or haemaccel, or concentrated red blood cells.

(continued)

Mentor: What equipment will we require for setting up IV fluids?

Student nurse:The bag of fluids, the line it runs through and the venflon that takes the fluid into the patient's vein.

Mentor:Yes, the line is called an administration set (or 'giving set') and we will also require gloves and an alcohol wipe or similar, such as a 2% chlorhexidine wipe, used to clean the cannula port when attaching the line. We will need to check that the cannula is patent before we attach it, which means that we will need to do a saline flush to make sure that the venflon is not blocked. We will also need to check for any problems with the patient's vein, such as pain and phlebitis, which we discussed earlier today.

Student nurse: Why do you wear gloves?

Mentor: An aseptic 'non-touch' technique is performed when administering IV fluids to reduce the chance of introducing germs into the patient's system. Gloves are also worn to reduce the chance of absorbing any antibiotics or other drugs that have been added to the fluid bag through our skin. We must always clean our hands before putting on our gloves, and when removing them too.

Mentor: What do you think are the main risks to the patient when administering IV fluids?

Student nurse: Like you said, introducing bugs into the patient's system.

Mentor: Some of the other risks when administering IV fluids are bacterial contamination, either local (phlebitis) or systemic (septic shock); speed shock; free flow; over- or under-infusion; inability to recall the drug and reverse the action of it and adverse reaction to the drug (if added to fluids, i.e. antibiotics).

Student nurse: What is speed shock?

Mentor: This is when drugs are administered too quickly and cause adverse effects, such as tinnitus in the case of the drug furosemide, the loop-diuretic drug.

Student nurse: What is a loop-diuretic drug?

Mentor: Diuretics make you go to the toilet more to pass urine. Patients often call these 'water pills' or even wrongly 'anti-water pills'. Drugs such as furosemide belong to a group of medicines known as loop-diuretics as they work on the loop of Henle in the kidneys. These drugs are prescribed to remove water in order to treat oedema (water retention) due to heart failure and can also be used to treat hypertension (high blood pressure). It would be good if you could read up on this area of the kidneys, to assist your understanding.

Mentor: When we administer IV drugs, it is important to deliver the fluid at the correct flow rate. If possible, use a pump to regulate the flow of infusion, but if no pump is available the drip rate must be calculated to deliver the correct amount over the correct time span. We would never administer blood or products with added potassium without a pump. Next time we are on a shift together I want you to tell me why this is.

Student nurse: OK. What changes the flow rate?

Mentor: The position of limb, the height of bag from the patient's shoulder and kinking of the tubing or cannula occlusion. Also, if the patient is very cold or very warm.

(continued)

Student nurse: How do you work out the correct flow rate if you don't have a machine or pump that works it out for you?

Mentor: Well, first you need to remember that we use two different types of administration set. One is for clear fluids; standard non-filtered giving set delivers 20 drops per millilitre. In contrast, a blood administration set has a filter. A blood giving set delivers 15 drops per millilitre. We can also use a burette in paediatric nursing, which delivers 60 drops per millilitre. This is the formula we use:

$$\text{Drip rate (in drops per minute)} = \frac{\text{Volume to be infused (mL)}}{\text{Time in hours}} \times \frac{\text{Drip rate}}{\text{Minutes per hour (60)}}$$

Let's look at an example. The doctor has prescribed 1 litre of sodium chloride 0.9% to be given over 8 hours:

$$\frac{1000 \text{ mL}}{8 \text{ hours}} \times \frac{20 \text{ drops per mL}}{60 \text{ min}} = 41.66$$

As we can't count 0.66 of a drop, we round this up to 42 drops per minute. The roller clamp on the administration line helps to slow down or speed up the flow rate. The drops per minute are counted in the chamber. I have a sheet I prepared for the last student I was mentoring: would you like one? Then next time you can prime the tubing after watching me perform the task now.

Student nurse: Yes, please. Thank you.

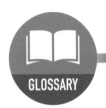

Phlebitis

Inflammation of a vein when a cannula is *in situ*. Regular monitoring of the intravenous access site is important.

Loop of Henle

Part of a small filter system – nephron – situated in the kidneys, responsible for filtering solutes, helping to maintain the correct balance of water in the body.

Box 12.1 Procedure for preparing intravenous fluids

- Collect all equipment.
- Wash your hands.
- If giving antibiotic therapy, gloves must be worn (sterile gloves are not required).
- Two checkers are required for IV therapy.
- Apply aseptic principles. Put on gloves.
- Check that you have the correct patient and gain consent.
- Inspect the fluid bag to be certain it contains the correct fluid, the fluid is clear (if the medication should be), the bag is not leaking and that the bag has not passed its use-by date.
- Sterile packaging must not be damaged or wet.
- Ensure that the correct giving set is being used for the fluid to be administered, as different sets are required for blood and blood products and electronic devices. These sets are either microdrip sets, which deliver 60 drops per millilitre into the drip chamber, or macrodrip sets, which deliver 15–20 drops per millilitre into the drip chamber.
- Open the packaging and uncoil the tubing. Do not let the ends of the tubing become contaminated. Close the flow regulator (roll the wheel away from the end you will attach the fluid bag).
- Remove the protective covering from the port of the fluid bag and the protective covering from the spike of the administration set.
- Insert the spike of the administration set into the port of the fluid bag with a quick twist. Do this carefully. Be especially careful not to puncture

(continued)

yourself! Insert the spike fully into the infusion bag, as there is an infection risk if it is not done properly.

- Hold the fluid bag higher than the drip chamber of the administration set. Squeeze the drip chamber once or twice to start the flow. Fill the drip chamber to one-third full. If you overfill the chamber, lower the bag below the level of the drip chamber and squeeze some fluid back into the fluid bag.

- Open the flow regulator and allow the fluid to flush all the air from the tubing. Let it run into the giving set empty packaging or container. You may need to loosen or remove the cap at the end of the tubing to get the fluid to flow to the end of the tubing (but this should not be necessary), taking care not to let the tip of the administration set become contaminated.

- The primed giving set is now ready to be connected to a electronic device, or the rate can be determined by gravity flow together with the flow clamp.

- Connect end of tubing to the patient: the intravenous cannula must be of an appropriate size for the intended use and cleaned with an alcohol and 2% chlorhexidine wipe before the giving-set end is attached, again to minimize infection risk. Wash your hands.

NOTE: aseptic technique must be adhered to throughout all intravenous procedures.

EXAMPLE: DRUG INTERACTIONS

Here is an example of a mentor–student learning-in-practice teaching session on drug interactions in psychiatry (Figure 12.2).

Daniel, a student nurse, has just completed his mental health placement and is puzzled as to why a patient suffering from severe depression had been told to avoid caffeine. All his mentor had told him was that this was because the patient was taking an 'MAOI'. When the patient had asked Daniel why he should avoid caffeine, Daniel said that he did not know. Daniel has no idea what an MAOI even was!

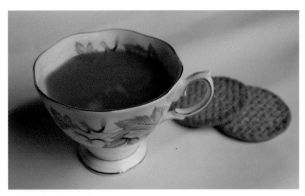

Figure 12.2 Drug interactions

Student nurse: Until recently when I looked this up, I had no idea what an MAOI was. I now know that this is a broad group of antidepressants known as monoamine oxidase inhibitors. These drugs work by balancing neurotransmitter chemicals in the brain to treat depression. I also found out that patients on these medications, such as phenelzine or tranylcypromine, have to avoid food and drinks that contain tyramine. What is tyramine?

Mentor: Sorry to hear your last mentor was not very helpful. Tyramine is found in foods such as strong, aged or processed cheeses, yogurt, sour cream (but not cream or ice cream), beef and chicken liver, dry sausage (such as salami, pepperoni), caviar, dried or pickled herring, anchovies and meats prepared with tenderisers. It is also in avocados, bananas, tinned figs, dried fruits, raspberries, overripe fruit, sauerkraut, soy beans, soy sauce, yeast extract, broad beans and excessive amounts of chocolate. Many foods and drinks with caffeine also contain tyramine, which is why your patient was informed that these drinks are best avoided while on this medication. Many alcoholic drinks also contain

(continued)

tyramine, such as red wine, draught beer and liqueurs. Non-alcoholic drinks and reduced-alcohol beers may also contain tyramine.

Student nurse: But what does tyramine do? Why should food and drink containing it be avoided?

Mentor: Tyramine reacts with MAOIs and may produce a large, sudden increase in blood pressure, known as hypertensive crisis.

Student nurse: Crikey! How would we know a patient on these medications was experiencing a hypertensive crisis?

Mentor: One of the first signs may be a throbbing headache.

Student nurse: Thank you. Now if a patient asks for information on MAOIs and tyramine I can explain.

Mentor: Why don't you look at the *British National Formulary*? It has a very good section on MAOIs.

Student nurse: Yes, I will.

TEST YOUR KNOWLEDGE

When you are next on clinical placement with your mentor, identify a learning need and ask your mentor to go through the clinical skill with you. Don't forget to get your assessment competencies signed off.

KEY POINTS

- What is bedside teaching?
- What are the benefits of bedside teaching?
- Effective learning in practice teaching
- Examples of teaching by learning in practice

Bibliography

Boyd, C. (2013) *Clinical Skills for Nurses*. Wiley Blackwell, Oxford.

British National Formulary (2013) *British National Formulary No. 66*. British Medical Association and Royal Pharmaceutical Society of Great Britain, London.

Cox, K. (1993) Planning bedside teaching. *Medical Journal of Australia* 158, 280–282.

Gill, D. (2007) *Teaching and Learning 'At the Bedside'*. Learning resource. Royal Free and University College Medical School, London.

Harth, S.C., Bavanandon, S., Thomas, K.E., Lai, M.Y. and Thong, Y.H. (1992) The quality of student–tutor interactions in the clinical learning environment. *Medical Education* 26, 321–326.

Nursing and Midwifery Council (2002) *An NMC Guide for Students of Nursing and Midwifery – Protecting the Public Through Professional Standards*. NMC, London.

Nursing and Midwifery Council (2008) *The Code: Standards of Conduct, Performance and Ethics for Nurses and Midwives*. NMC, London; www.nmc-uk.org/code.

Nursing and Midwifery Council (2011) *The Prep Handbook*. NMC, London; www.nmc-uk.org.

Chapter 13

MINIMISING
STRESS

Study Skills for Nurses, First Edition. Claire Boyd and contributing author, Beverley Murray
© 2014 John Wiley & Sons, Ltd. Published 2014 by John Wiley & Sons Ltd.

LEARNING OUTCOMES

By the end of this chapter you will have an understanding of the effects of stress on the body and strategies to minimise these effects.

Certain words in our vocabulary instil fear in the human spirit like no others. These words depend on the individual but common ones bringing many of us out in a cold sweat are 'deadline' and 'examination date'! Throughout your training there will be many times when you feel overwhelmed with your university work, your placement and events in your personal life. Your nursing course is not just about university results, but also about your future and your career, adding extra pressure with assessments as well as examinations and assignments.

Organising your study can minimise stress; conversely, leaving your study to the very last minute and being unprepared may increase it. However, many people need the added pressure for motivation, when time is against them. Key control measures to minimise stress involve being organised, looking after your health and using strategies for relaxation.

To experience some stress in our daily lives is actually a good thing. It is only when this stress takes control and overpowers us that it can start to affect our health. Working in health care can be very physical, and we need to be in tip-top form. It is important to be aware of the effects of stress on health and well-being.

HEALTH

Good health has three main elements. They are:

- social health (often referred to as socioeconomic health),
- physical health,
- psychological health.

Table 13.1 Examples of detriments to the elements of health

Health element	Example
Physical	Someone has an accident at work and is unable to work anymore. Loses job.
Social	Income severely curtailed and unable to pay bills. Falls into debt. Also unable to afford good nutrition, so immune system is weakened and person is prone to illness.
Psychological	Becomes depressed.

An example of each (see Table 13.1) shows how all these factors are interrelated.

The phenomemon of **stress** is also a good example of how these factors are all interrelated. It has been suggested that there is only one way to avoid stress, and that is to die! Therefore stress is an inevitable part of our lives, affecting everyone.

THE STRESS RESPONSE

The **stress response** or **fight-or-flight response** is when our bodies are flooded with adrenaline and other hormones, which prompt a number of alert responses. These include faster heart rate and heightened muscle tension, allowing us to respond quickly to the danger or *stressor* present.

For most people stress is negative, such as stressful life events (e.g. family problems or financial problems). But too little stress can cause feelings of listlessness and under-stimulation, resulting in slow and inefficient performance, or even depression. We have all seen an athlete who is about to run an important race getting pumped up before the start. The athlete needs **positive stress** to perform well. However, we need equilibrium: a good balance of this negative and positive stress.

With too much negative stress – when stressor is piled upon stressor – our bodies become unable to maintain balance (homeostasis) between encounters, which may be life-threatening. An example of this is when the body continues to manufacture stress chemicals over a prolonged period and the immune system becomes depressed and functions poorly. The effects of high stress levels on the body and our behaviour, thoughts, emotions and health can be seen.

RELAXATION

One way to reduce negative stress is to find ways to relax. However, something may be relaxing for one individual and quite stressful for another. There are a number of ways an person can obtain a state of relaxation, often after practice. These include meditation, visualisation, guided imagery and progressive muscular relaxation, known as PMR (Friedman 1974). Activity 13.1 shows how to perform the PMR exercise.

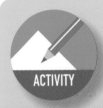

Activity 13.1

ACTIVITY

Here is the procedure for progressive muscular relaxation, or the relaxation muscle tense-and-release system.

Put on some soothing music on low volume. Lie comfortably on the floor, with a cushion under your head for support, in a quiet room. Remove your shoes. You can start at the head and face or toes. Perform the exercise slowly, working through each tense-and-release section. This exercise will take approximately 20 minutes to perform.

1   Focus on your breathing. Slowly breathe in, in, in and out. Emphasise the out breath. Take a few more breaths before moving on.
2   Tense the muscles in your right foot, hold for a few seconds, then release. Tense and release the calf muscle, then the thigh muscles (tense and release). Repeat with the left foot and leg.
3   Tense and release the muscles in your right hand. Tense and release the muscles in your right arm. Then the left hand and arm.

4   Tense and release each buttock. Then the stomach muscles.
5   Lift your shoulders up to your ears, hold for a few seconds, then lower.
     Repeat three times. Rock your head gently from side to side.
6   Yawn, then pout. Frown, wrinkle your nose and let go. Raise your
     eyebrows then relax your face muscles.
7   Focus on your breathing again. Wriggle your fingers and toes, bend your
     knees and gently roll over on to your side. Get up slowly.

Simpler ways for a moment's peace of mind may include a soak in a lovely bath, listening to music and my husbands' particular favourite, the biophilia hypothesis (although he did not know it!). The biophilia hypothesis was devised by Edward Wilson, who suggested that the brain is 'hardwired' to nature and the reason why people need to 'touch base' with the sea, forests and the open countryside. In short, humans have an 'innate affinity with nature' (Wilson 1984) (Figure 13.1). This is why GPs may suggest that patients

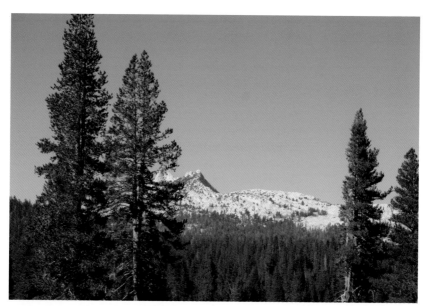

Figure 13.1 Getting back to nature

go for a walk in the country to alleviate the symptoms of stress and depression and it is also the rationale for having flowers in our houses and in hospital: it cheers people up. Many hospital environments now no longer allow flowers at the bedside due to infection control and health and safety (water spillage).

GLOSSARY

Physiological
Pertaining to the physical body.

When someone is ill, there is a tendency to treat the ailment (known as the medical approach). But due to the fact that all bodily systems are interlinked it has long been recognised (Westwood 2001) that a 'holistic' approach should be sought, treating the 'whole person' (the biopsychosocial approach). Over a long period of time stress can have a negative impact on the body, causing a vast array of physiological problems, such as raised blood pressure and suppression of the immune system due to the increased cortisol levels which are known to decrease numbers of white blood cells such as lymphocytes. The stress response also causes the thymus to become less effective, therefore decreasing the number of antibodies produced. Without antibodies the immune system is severely weakened and the body's ability to fight infection is reduced, increasing the number of colds and other illnesses experienced. In addition, the body can become more susceptible to immune-system-related diseases such as rheumatoid arthritis, allergies, asthma and – research suggests – even cancer (Looker and Gregson 2003). It therefore follows that relaxation is beneficial to the body, reducing the amount of negative stress an individual experiences.

Relaxation therapy allows the immune system to recover and to function more effectively. It lowers blood pressure, therefore decreasing the likelihood of experiencing a stroke and/or heart attack. The brain has a regular need for more pronounced right-hemispheric activity (the calming part of the brain) and relaxation helps to meet this need (Elliott 2008).

NUTRITION

During times of stress the body's demand for 'fuel' increases, and therefore nutrition plays an important part in the relaxation process. So, make sure you eat properly, keeping to a well-balanced diet. Supplements such as vitamin tablets may be taken to replenish the body's demand for these increased resources, restoring health. Coffee, smoking and alcohol all contribute to feelings of stress, whereas physical exercise can help to decrease levels in some people.

BREATHING

Another physiological element of the stress response is to change the breathing pattern, often leading to a shallow and rapid breathing pattern, utlising mainly the upper part of the thorax. Insufficient oxygen is inhaled and carbon dioxide builds up in the bloodstream, making the blood more acidic. Over time, this lack of oxygen to the vital organs becomes apparent, with individuals perhaps yawning initially, then experiencing dizziness, confusion, headache, tiredness and lack of concentration. Over a period of time this breathing pattern become the norm and it is for this reason that deep-breathing exercises are often recommended as a means of correcting this and initiating a state of wellness.

This chapter has shown how the biopsychosocial elements of all individuals are interlinked. By reducing the sympathetic nervous system activity physiological parameters can be brought within the normal range; this can be achieved through relaxation treatments.

VISUALISING

To decrease your stress levels when on an academic course, such as nursing, strategies can be implemented to achieve a 'quick fix'. One of my favourite strategies is finding a quiet place and visualising: removing myself far from the here and now, and taking myself off to some exotic paradise.

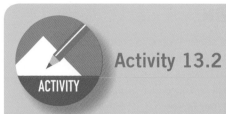

Activity 13.2

This is the five-senses imagery exercise.

Spend 50 seconds imagining each item. Better still, get someone to read this list to you while you lie down and close your eyes. The whole exercise should take only approximately 5 minutes.

- **Sight** Visualize a palm tree, full of lush green leaves. See it.
- **Sound** Think of complete darkness. Imagine the sound of waves lapping against a shore. Listen to seagulls in the sky. Hear it.
- **Smell** Conjure up the smell of fresh, salty sea air. Smell it.
- **Taste** Visualize a lemon. Look at its shape and colour. Slice it in the middle and look at the fresh, juicy glistening flesh. Squeeze it gently and let the juice drip. Take the cut end to your mouth and lick it. Taste it.
- **Touch** Evoke the tactile image of walking barefoot over warm, soft sand on a hot summer's day. Feel it.
- **Kinaesthetic sense (perception of body movement)** Lastly, feel yourself engaged in the activity of climbing a sand dune. Imagine it.

ORGANISATION

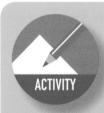

Activity 13.3

Photocopy the year planner at the back of this book and write down all your shifts. Write down days you are to attend university and submission dates for assignments, etc. In short, get organised.

Nothing will cut down your stress levels like getting organised. Look at the year planner at the back of this book and use this not only for your shifts but also for your assignments, submission dates and other important events. Organise your workload. This should be very helpful. Review Chapter 3 for further tips on organising your workload.

SOURCES OF SUPPORT

Sometimes things will get on top of you, and in such times do not be afraid to seek support. Often, just talking things through with someone else can help the situation, be it your tutor, your mentor, a peer, someone from the university counselling service or someone from the student services department or student union. You may choose to use a social media forum for assistance.

Lastly, it is important to take regular breaks away from your study. However, personally I don't like the stop-and-start approach and prefer longer stints or work. Fin what works for you. Don't forget to enjoy your course and have some fun, but keep to those deadlines!

TEST YOUR KNOWLEDGE

1   What are the three elements that make up the biopsychosocial approach to health?
2   What is the biopsychosocial approach to health also known as?
3   What is the biophilia hypothesis?
4   Lie down on a comfortable bed. Now visualise yourself on a tropical beach, listening to the waves lapping against the shore. The sun is in a cloudless sky. Just relax. Take long deep breaths.

KEY POINTS

- The biopsychosocial approach to health
- The stress response
- Getting organised
- Quick-fix relaxation technique

Bibliography

Elliott, R. (2008) *The Truth About Relaxation Techniques, Seminar Notes.* Ohio State University, USA.

Friedman, M. (1974) *Type A Behaviour; it's Diagnosis and Treatment.* Plenum, London.

Looker, T. and Gregson, O. (2003) *Teach Yourself; Managing Stress.* Hodder & Stoughton, London.

McGuinness, H. (2000) *Indian Head Massage.* Bookpoint, Oxford.

Westwood, C. (2001) *Stress Management – a Guide for Home Use.* Amberwood Publishing, Guildford.

Wilson, E. (1984) *Biophilia.* Harvard University Press, Cambridge, MA.

Answers to Activities and Test Your Knowledge

CHAPTER 1

Activity 1.1

Lecture	Large groups (could be over 100 students) all coming together for a teaching session. You will need to take notes, but you may also be given handouts of the teaching session.
Seminar	This is usually groups of up to 30 with one tutor. The emphasis is on group discussions. Students may also be asked to prepare presentations to the group.
Tutorial	Group sizes vary from one student to anything up to 15. Tutorials often focus on one particular topic or assignment. They can also be a chance to 'touch base' with your personal tutor to see how your clinical placements are going. Personal tutorials are usually one-to-one and can also concern pastoral issues.
Practicals	These may involve workshops and give you the chance to work on a practical level. This may mean going to a clinical skills laboratory to learn how to perform observations, make beds, perform bed baths, etc. Practicals provide the opportunity to learn skills you will need in clinical placement.
Self-guided study	This is where students work through prepared materials, which may be on paper or computer based (they can include audio or video media). This form of study may be referred to as distance learning.
Computer-aided learning	Computers are part of the twenty-first century and are used to support the learning process. Computers can take the student through a teaching programme and can be used in such activities as maths revision.

(continued)

Study Skills for Nurses, First Edition. Claire Boyd and contributing author, Beverley Murray
© 2014 John Wiley & Sons, Ltd. Published 2014 by John Wiley & Sons Ltd.

Assessment	Assessments help to maintain standards and allows levels of achievement to be recognised. Throughout your training you will be given competency assessment documentation for you to grade your own performance and for your mentor/preceptor to assess your ability, e.g. in drug administration.

Activity 1.2

1 Excellent people skills
2 Good communication and observation
3 Ability to answer questions and offer advice
4 Happy to work as part of a team
5 Be able to deal with emotionally charged situations

Activity 1.3

application	A program running on a computer that does a particular job, e.g. web browser or word processor.
attachment	A file attached to an email message. It could be a picture or a document.
broadband	A fast telephone connection designed mainly for computer use.
browser	A program, such as Internet Explorer, that allows you look at web pages.
compact disc (CD)	A disc that can be used to store information.
download	The process of moving a file from a remote system, such as a server, to your personal computer.
file	A collection of information stored under one name; may be a document, spreadsheet or picture.
firewall	A security system on a computer which controls incoming and outgoing information.
folder	A group of files held together in one place. Folders can contain other folders within them.
forum	This is an online meeting place, much like a public notice board. Members of the forum can send and reply to messages.
gigabyte (GB)	A measurement of data size or storage capacity; approximately equivalent to 1000 megabytes (MB), 1 million kilobytes (kB) or 1 billion bytes.

hard disc	A disc that is usually fitted inside the computer (but not always) which holds large quantities of information.
input device	Hardware used to communicate with your computer, such as a mouse and keyboard.
internet	The vast collection of interconnected computers throughout the world that can exchange information and communicate with each other.
Internet Explorer (IE)	A web browser program, made by Microsoft.
ISP (internet service provider)	A company that provides for access to the internet (often charges for this service).
megabyte (MB)	A measurement of data size or storage capacity; approximately 1 million bytes.
modem	A device that links the computer to the internet.
memory	The part of your computer where the data is stored.
operating system	The master program that controls your computer, such as Microsoft Windows. It is what you use to give your computer instructions.
output device	Hardware that a computer uses to communicate with you, such as screen and speakers.
portable document format (PDF)	A common file format defined by Adobe Systems, used to create documents that you can read. You will require PDF reader software to read these files.
processor	The device in a computer that performs all the work.
program	The instructions that tell a computer what to do. May also be called software or an application. Programs can be installed from a disc or by downloading from the internet.
RAM memory	The active memory of a computer: it's the bit the does the work, but it doesn't store anything. More RAM makes your computer faster.
router	Hardware that can be used to set up a wireless network in your home by distributing internet connections to one or more computers.
software	The common term for computer programs or applications.

(continued)

spam	Unsolicited and unwanted email.
uniform resource locator (URL)	An address that identifies the location of a website. Also known as a web address.
universal serial bus (USB)	A socket into which you can plug equipment like a printer, web camera or USB flash drive.
USB flash drive	A small, portable memory device that can be plugged into a USB socket. May also be known as a memory stick, pen drive or disgo.
virus	A program that can damage part of your computer. Designed to replicate itself.
web	A collection of web pages on the internet, accessible through a web browser. Can also be used to refer to the internet.
web browser	A program that allows you to look at web pages, such as Internet Explorer.
wireless fidelity (WiFi)	A wireless technology that allows computers to communicate without the need for any physical connection between them. WiFi are more commonly found on laptop computers.
window	A box outlined on your screen showing one activity or program. You can have a number of windows open at one time.
Windows	The most common operating system found on personal computers; made by Microsoft.

Adapted from Open University (2011).

Chapter 1 Test Your Knowledge

The answer will be personal to you.

CHAPTER 2

Activity 2.1

The text is actually a shorthand abbreviation giving you information from the 2001 UK Census:

Between **1991** and **2001** there had been a **53**% growth in the minority ethnic population.

(From 3.0 million in 1991 to 4.6 million in 2001.)

Activity 2.2

Starting with the first letter of the alphabet, 'a', an 'o' has been added after each letter in sequence until you got to 'f' then a 'p' has been added after each letter in sequence.

Activity 2.3

The pattern went: two tablets, four capsules, four capsules, two tablets, four capsules, four capsules, two tablets.

Activity 2.4

Visual learners: you may have used coloured highlighter pens to mark key words and sentences.

Audio learners: you may have read the text loud.

Kinaesthetic learners: you may have read the text while walking around.

Activity 2.5

Advantages of distance learning: helpful to students who are unable to get to a given location; students can proceed at their own pace; convenient; students may prefer this approach away from large groups.

Disadvantages of distance learning: can be expensive to design and produce; may not get instant tutor feedback or assistance; students may find it difficult to get and remain motivated; students may feel isolated; students may not get peer support.

Activity 2.6

Advantages of e-learning: helpful to students who are unable to get to a given location; students can proceed at their own pace; convenient, student may prefer this approach away from large groups.

Disadvantages of e-learning: can be expensive to design and produce; students may feel isolated; students may not get peer support; students need to have good IT skills.

Chapter 2 Test Your Knowledge

1   Your course handbook will contain details of all the student services. Universities also have 'one-stop' shops for information. You may also need to speak to your personal tutor.

2   **(a)** Change grams into kilograms:
$975/1000 = 0.975 \ (0.98)$
Then use the weight formula to see how much of the drug the baby required according to body weight: weight (kg) × dose:
0.975×15 mg
$= 14.625$ mg

   (b) weight (kg) × dose, 1.8 kg
$\times 5$ mg $= 9$ mg

   (c) i weight (kg) × dose, 4.2 kg
$\times 50$ mg $= 210$ mg

      ii volume of drug to be given
$= \dfrac{\text{what you want}}{\text{what you've got}} \times \text{volume}$
$\dfrac{210 \text{ mg}}{600 \text{ mg}} \times 4 \text{ mL} = 1.4 \text{ mL}$

   (d) weight (kg) × dose, 2.2 kg
$\times 0.4$ mg $= 0.88$ mg
It is given by intramuscular injection.

(e) Volume of drug to be given

$$= \frac{\text{what you want}}{\text{what you've got}} \times \text{volume}$$

$$\frac{40 \text{ mg}}{50 \text{ mg}} \times 2 \text{ mL} = 1.6 \text{ mL}$$

(f) **i** weight (kg) × dose, 3.1 kg
× 2 mg = 6.2 mg

ii 6.2 mg × 1000/50/3.1 kg
× 0.5 mL = 20 mcg/kg/h

(g) **i** weight (kg) × dose, 3.1 kg
× 120 mg = 372 mg

ii 372 mg × 1000/50/3.1 kg/
60 × 0.25 mL/h
= 10 mcg/kg/min

CHAPTER 3

Activity 3.1

Speak to the person concerned: are they having any difficulties with their allocated task? Why do you feel unfairly treated? Speak to other groups: how did they manage this situation? Speak to your personal tutor, the tutor concerned with the task or a student counsellor. Remember, the responsibility for the group lies with each member of it. Every member shares responsibility for sorting out the problem so that the group can achieve its purpose and not blame one person.

Chapter 3 Test Your Knowledge

See table at bottom of the page.

CHAPTER 4

Chapter 4 Test Your Knowledge

1 Patient or population, Intervention or exposure, Comparisons, Outcome(s)

2 Title and abstract, abstract, author, ISSN number, journal name, publication type, title, any field

3 Date, article and publication types, human or animal, gender, age groups, language

4 To keep words in together in a phrase

MONTH: October	Monday	Tuesday	Wednesday	Thursday	Friday	Sat	Sun
Week 1	Mtg with personal tutor at 2 pm, between Uni lectures	Meet with support group to discuss ethics essay, after Uni lectures Social media to discuss ethics	Planning: ethics essay Read ethics lecture notes before work	Go to library: literature search, ethics: before work Mtg with mentor to go through competencies to be signed off	Go to library: literature search, ethics: after work	Washing, shopping Nocte: Brad's party Buy Mum's birthday present	Start to prepare draft ethics essay
Work shift	Uni	Uni	Late shift	Late shift	Early shift	Day off	Day off

5 Allow for variations in word endings

6 Take into account different spelling variations

7 AND, OR, NOT

8 AND and NOT

9 OR

10 Yes

CHAPTER 5

Activity 5.4

1 Three. The question did not ask you to name them (hyaline cartilage, hyaline yellow elastic cartilage and hyaline white fibrocartilage).

2 Lungs, walls of arteries, trachea and bronchial tubes.

3 To transport oxygen and food to all cells, fight infection and to make clots.

4 Erythrocytes, leucocytes, thrombocytes, plasma.

Activity 5.5

1 Check your course notes: should the text have been double spaced?

2 Check your course notes: should the text have been produced in Times New Roman?

3 *Individuals* does not need an apostrophe, as it is not possessive

4 *Stereotyping* spelt wrongly.

5 Should be *In* the *nursing profession....*

6 *personal* reflection

7 there are six major *categories...*

8 general *public*

9 have been *receiving*

10 extremely *problematic*

Chapter 5 Test Your Knowledge

1 Non-passive reading; extracting all the information from the text; purposeful reading

2 Survey, question, read, recall, review

3 See table below:

Connective tissue	Structure	Function	Location
Areolar	Elastic, allowing high degree of movement Can also allow fluids to pass through	Connecting and supporting other tissues, e.g. binds skin to muscles	Between skin and muscles, supporting blood vessels and nerves in alimentary canal
Adipose	Made up of a large amount of fat cells	White: support, protection, insulating layer; also food reserve Brown: helps to retain heat; energy store	White: eyes, kidneys, between muscles and under skin Brown: walls of large blood vessels, trunk, nape of neck; between scapulae

(continued)

Connective tissue	Structure	Function	Location
Lymphoid	Semi-solid tissue	Lymphocyte cells engulf and destroy bacteria	Found in lymph nodes, thymus, the spleen, tonsils, wall of large intestine, appendix, glands of small intestine
Yellow elastic	Elastic fibres capable of considerable extension and recoil	To enable stretch and recoil of organs and vessels	Lung tissue, walls of arteries, trachea (wind pipe) bronchial tubes
White fibrous	Little elasticity, collagen fibres run in same direction	Connection and protection to parts of the body	Skin (dermis), ligaments (tendons), cartilage and bones
Bone (osseous tissue)	Hardest tissue in the body, next to the teeth	To support and protect body and all its organs; to produce blood cells in bone marrow	Two types: Compact: dense bone for strength Cancellous: structure-bearing and cellular development = skeleton
Vascular tissue	Blood: connective tissue Erythrocytes, leucocytes, thrombocytes, plasma	To transport oxygen and food to all cells, fights infection and form clots	All over body
Hyaline cartilage	Most common type of cartilage, particularly resilient	Protection, provides flexibility, supports and aids movement of joints	Costal cartilages (connects ribs to sternum), parts of larynx, trachea, bronchi, nose and end of bones which forms joints
Hyaline yellow elastic cartilage	Elastic fibres distributed in a solid matrix	Flexibility, maintains shape and gives support	Found in parts of the body that move freely: the pinnae, part of the wall of blood vessels, Eustachian tubes, epiglottis

Connective tissue	Structure	Function	Location
Hyaline white fibrocartilage	Tough bundle of dense white fibres, slightly flexible	To absorb shock	Disc between vertebrae, pad between the knee joint bones, hip, shoulder sockets and pubic symphysis

4 There are no errors!
5 Qualitative/quantitative/mixed-methods research
6 Comprehensive, comparison, interpretation, analysis, evaluation

CHAPTER 6

Activity 6.1

& and
+ in addition, plus
> greater or more than
< smaller or less than
= equal to or same as
w/ with
→ this leads to/produces/causes

Activity 6.2

STAT immediately
AC *ante cibum* (before food)
BD *bis die* (twice daily)
OD *omni die* (every day)
OM *omni mane* (every morning)
ON *omni nocte* (every night)
PC *post cibum* (after food)
PRN *pro re nata* (when required)
QDS *quarter die sumendus* (to be taken four times daily)
QQH *quarta quaque hora* (every 4 hours)
TDS *ter die sumendus* (to be taken three times daily)
TID *ter in die* (three times daily)

Activity 6.3

The notes from this lecture look more like an essay! The student did not use any short-hand or abbreviations such as &. Even 'maternal deprivation' was written in full each time, instead of 'MD'. Figures were written in words; i.e. 'five' instead of '5'. The whole lecture notes were written in long-hand instead of a note format. Much of the lecture would not have been heard as the student would have been so focused on writing down each word that the lecturer was saying.

The first two sections could be written as:

> Montrophy (MT) = become attached to one figure
>
> Imprinting = rapid form of attachment – develop BOND
>
> Bowlby (BW) 1951 – human infants form special bond with mother – known as MT, similar to imprinting

Look again at the lecture notes and see how you would condense them.

Activity 6.4

1 Flow chart of notifiable disease process:

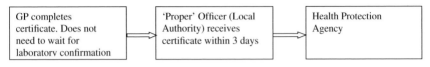

| GP completes certificate. Does not need to wait for laboratory confirmation | → | 'Proper' Officer (Local Authority) receives certificate within 3 days | → | Health Protection Agency |

2 Spider diagram of notifiable diseases:

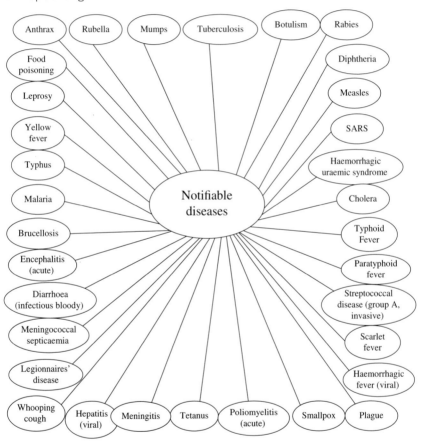

The idea of a flow diagram is to put one piece of information in boxes and to show movement of a process using arrows between the boxes. A spider diagram is a good way to record the notifiable diseases, but a flow diagram is good for recording the notifiable disease process.

Chapter 6 Test Your Knowledge

Spider diagram with *urinalysis* in the centre, with lines radiating out to the terms *blood*, *pH*, *bilirubin*, *ketones*, *nitrites*, *glucose*, *leucocytes* and *protein*.

Remember you were not asked to record any more details other that what urinalysis detects.

CHAPTER 7

Activity 7.1

1 Copying
2 Failing to reference direct quotes from a source
3 Paraphrasing or synthesising
4 Using your own previous work without acknowledging this as the case

Activity 7.2

Well, clearly student 2 has committed plagiarism, not using any references and copying the main text. Plagiarism may not always be quite so clear cut; your note-taking must be in your own words, which will remove any chance of you committing plagiarism by directly 'lifting' someone else's work, as this student has clearly done.

Chapter 7 Test Your Knowledge

1 Plagiarism is using someone else's work, words, ideas or thinking and failing to reference or give credit to that person when you have used any of this in your own work.
2 An alphabetical list, arranged by author surname, listing the sources of information that you have used as background reading.
3 A list of sources that *you have cited* in your assignment. This may be arranged alphabetically by author surname (Harvard system) or numbered (Vancouver system).
4 Autonomy, beneficence, fidelity, justice, non-maleficence, veracity

CHAPTER 8

Activity 8.1

Relevance	The perceived relevance to health care
Supervision	The availability of tutors to supervise and the willingness of other health carers to help you with your dissertation
Interest	Your existing knowledge of the topic and the strength of your desire to learn more about it
Competence	Your skill at employing proposed methods of data collection and data analysis
Scale	The feasibility of completing the study within the time available and with the resources at hand.

Adapted from Chandler (2012).

Chapter 8 Test Your Knowledge

1   The paragraphs are shown as in the text below.

> **An investigation into the incidents and effects of hospital induced malnutrition on adult patients undergoing non-minor surgical procedures.**
>
> This assignment will explore the incidence and effects of hospital induced malnutrition (HIM) on adult patients undergoing non-minor surgical procedures, such as an appendicectomy.
>
> An argument will be forwarded for the provision of nutrition assessment and continued monitoring (NACM) for surgical patients, with examples of assessment and monitoring tools in practice. An exploration of the financial cost to the National Health Service of non-assessment and monitoring will be further investigated.
>
> However, before proceeding, brief descriptions of the terms 'malnutrition' and 'nutritional assessment' would be deemed necessary. Malnutrition can be defined as an inadequate balance of dietary intake for health maintaining requirements (Oxford, 1991). It is recognised that some patients are malnourished on admission to hospital, however, for the purpose of this assignment, only HIM will be explored. Nutritional assessment can be divided into two sections – an assessment of nutritional status and assessment of nutrient intake i.e. continued monitoring (Reilly, 1996), usually performed by questioning, observation and body mass index (BMI) calculations.
>
> Whilst on clinical placement, a thirty-two year old otherwise fit and healthy male was admitted to hospital with suspected appendicitis. After undergoing an appendicectomy, Richard (a pseudonym) made a poor recovery (lethargic etc.). After clinical investigation (serum proteins, anthropometric evaluations), it transpired that Richard was malnourished. It seemed incredible that a patient in 1996, in a modern hospital had experienced HIM – rationale prompting an investigation into the incidence and effects of malnutrition on otherwise healthy surgical patients. Investigations showed that Richard's experience of malnutrition was far from an isolated incidence: Moynihan (1994) states that malnutrition was far from an isolated incidence: Moynihan

(1994) states that malnutrition in surgical patients is regarded as a 'common problem' with 40 – 50% of these patients showing signs of malnutrition following surgery, due to the associated trauma of the surgery increasing the need for nutrients, specifically proteins used for the repair of body tissue (Andrewes et al, 1994).

Personal experience from clinical practice has shown that nutritional assessment is performed on patients as part of the admission procedure at a very basic level, whereby patients are questioned about their usual appetite and ability to eat and swallow. Patients deemed to be at a high risk of developing malnutrition are then weighed and usually referred to the dietician. However, this basic assessment would appear to be very ineffective due to the high incidence of malnutrition post-operatively (as discussed previously). Andrewes et al (1994) states that an effective nutritional assessment should contain twelve question/factors, such as 'appetite' and 'needs related illness' (Appendix 1). Bacon (1996) further suggests that nurses in the front line should initiate a thorough assessment on all patients, with a multidisciplinary approach with referrals to the Dietician where appropriate. It can therefore be suggested that a nutritional assessment could be incorporated. It can therefore be suggested that a nutritional assessment could be incorporated with the full admission procedures, with minimal increase of time.

Nutritional assessment also involves continued monitoring to assess exactly what the patient has eaten. A good tool for this purpose is the food chart whereby all food consumed is accurately documented thereby identifying potential problems, such as inadequate intake.

Bacon (1996) states that the food chart is as valuable as a fluid chart and should be completed with the same degree of accuracy. By incorporating this continued monitoring on patients throughout their hospital stay would hi-light patients with insufficient dietary intake, such as Richard, whose malnutrition had stemmed from a dislike of the food on offer. Patients otherwise fit and healthy as Richard on admission would not be considered a 'high risk' and may slip through the net becoming malnourished post-operatively.

(continued)

It can therefore be argued that all patients undergoing surgical procedures should be nutritionally assessed pre-operatively with on-going continued monitoring post-operatively with the use of food charts and patient weighing, thereby picking up abnormalities of nutritional status before becoming problematic (Reilly, 1996).

The rationale for this NACM on surgical patients is due to the fact that malnutrition among patients in hospital is often not recognised despite the serious clinical (Reilly, 1996, Appendix 2) and financial consequences (Norton, 1996). This is despite the fact that malnutrition prolongs recovery, increases the need for high-dependency nursing, increases the risk of serious complications of illness and increases the incidence of mortality (Davison, 1996). Non-monitoring of nutritional intake could prove to be fatal: Zainal (1995) estimates that in simple starvation, a weight loss of 39 – 40% can be fatal, but in the critically ill, a much lower weight loss may result in death. Holmes (1991) further states that without lower weight loss may result in death. Holmes (1991) further states that without nutritional support, even in previously 'normal' patients, such losses are accompanied by clinical effects which increase morbidity; nutritional assessment would have the effect of reducing the duration of disability, improving wound healing, lessening the incidence of complications and ultimately reducing mortality.

Charalambous (1993) states that during a prolonged hospital stay, malnutrition can often increase or develop for the first time. It is recognised that in-patients stay has been considerably reduced, with emphasis placed on 'care in the community' (as discussed by Alexander et al, 1994). However, it should be noted that patients such as Richard had not eaten for two/three days prior to admission due to pain and nausea, combined with the period of starvation and fluid deprivation prior to anaesthesia (as discussed by Bates, 1994), coupled with the trauma of surgery to bodily systems (Holmes, 1991) all combining to raise the possibility of malnutrition. Indicating, yet again, for the introduction of NACM on all surgical patients, not just those considered 'high risk' on admission.

To lower the incidence and identify patients at greater risk of developing HIM post-operatively, calculations of Body mass Index (BMI) may be initiated on admission, whereby the weight in Kilograms is divided by height in metres squared – normal range within the 20–22 region (Davidson, 1996). However, BMI does not give a true reflection of nutritional status (Pennington, 1994); weighing patients on admission followed by daily weights shows more clearly the degree of unintentional or inappropriate weight loss. Reilly (1996) states that the following equation may be used to give a clear indication of nutritional status:

$$\% \text{ Weight loss} = \frac{\text{Usual weight} - \text{actual weight}}{\text{Usual weight}} \times 100$$

A further method of lowering the incidence of HIM would be to provide diets for individual tastes and preferences. The Patient's Charter (1992) states that:

'You have a choice of dishes, including meals suitable for all dietary needs'.

However, Nazarko (1993) states that food should be appropriate for ethnic dietary needs, describing that some services often assume that the entire UK population follow a 'traditional British diet', therefore alienating this group of patients and potentially giving rise to the possibility of HIM – rationale for the training of catering staff and dieticians in special dietary requirements. A thorough assessment of all patients on admission should hi-light special dietary needs/requirements (as discussed previously).

It can be further argued that Richard became malnourished due to lack of communication and observation by nursing staff, rationale for the introduction of training programmes by dieticians. Further evidence for the introduction of NACM on surgical patients nutritional needs, and training of health personnel, can be found in the Kings Fund Report (1992, as cited by Harvey, 1993) which states a need to develop the 'recognition of under-nourishment' and to 'increase awareness' of situations in which they occur.

(continued)

This would seem especially important as Norton (1996) states that many Doctors and Nurses do not recognise the importance of monitoring patients' nutrition. Nurses are in the unique position of being able to nutritionally assess all patients being admitted as a routine part of the admission procedure, thereby giving more efficient use of resources by involving the dietician for those patients to be in need of nutritional intervention only.

The Department of Health (as cited by Holmes, 1994) recommended the assessment of nutritional status becoming routine for all 'older patients', however, it has been shown that vulnerability to malnutrition applies to all surgical patients. Harvey (1993) states that the actual nutritional requirements between young and older individuals varies little between these groups, only the **energy** requirements, further rationale for the introduction of NACM on all patients.

Holistic care involves the need for 'individualised nursing' focusing care around the unique needs of the individual (Henderson, 1982, as cited by Reed, 1992). Therefore dismissing sections of society such as the healthy adult on admission, and only performing nutritional assessment and monitoring on the elderly and those considered to be at highest risk could, if malnutrition becomes evident, be viewed as paramount to negligence, further reasoning for the introduction of NACM on all patients.

Malnutrition increases the cost of hospitalisation (Holmes, 1996) due to the delayed recovery. Charalambous (1993) states that if 10% of hospital in-patients had their stay reduced by five days as a result of better nutritional support, an estimated £266 million would be saved annually in the U.K. This figure does not incorporate the financial costs to the NHS of patient litigation for negligence. Therefore, it can be suggested, exceeding the cost of implementing nutritional assessment on every surgical patient. Nutritional assessment would appear to be very effective. Queen's Medical Centre perform a full nutritional assessment on every patient admitted to the medical directorate thus lowering the incidence of HIM (Field, 1995).

Routinely assessing every patient nutritionally would give the nurse the ideal opportunity to incorporate Health Education on healthy eating matters (as discussed by Health of the Nation (DOH, 1992), with a view to lowering the incidence of mortality due to unhealthy eating habits by a large proportion of the general public.

To conclude, this assignment has argued for the need to reduce the unacceptable levels of HIM by implementing the following factors:

- Nutritional Assessment and continued monitoring (NACM) on all non-minor surgical patients (to include daily weighing).
- Dieticians to raise awareness of special dietary needs, including ethic variations in diet.
- Nurses to be offered on-going training programmes regarding special nutritional needs of surgical patients.
- Nurses to be aware of and recognise the effect of malnourishment on patients and to become actively involved in eliminating the incidence of hospital induced malnutrition.

A multidisciplinary approach is recommended, with the incorporation of Health Education on assessment.

It is further suggested to audit the incidence of HIM on for an accurate, up-to-date picture of the cost of this to the NHS. It is hoped that the results of this audit may warrant initiating funding to incorporate the introduction of NACM on all surgical patients i.e. proving to be cost-effective.

Moynihan (1994) states that malnutrition in surgical patients is largely avoidable: By incorporating NACM on surgical patients, HIM may be largely eliminated and patients may experience the high quality care to which they are entitled and to which they expect.

CHAPTER 9

Chapter 9 Test Your Knowledge

I would prepare a poster to help with this presentation, showing a commode and all the areas that need to be cleaned, adding important information around cleaning products.

No infection – clean all areas as indicated with detergent wipes.

Infection or Outbreak – clean with Actichlor 1000ppm
(1 tablet in 1 litre of cold water)

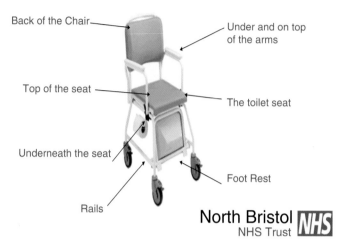

Back of the Chair

Under and on top
of the arms

Top of the seat

The toilet seat

Underneath the seat

Foot Rest

Rails

North Bristol **NHS**
NHS Trust

Source: North Bristol NHS Trust and University Hospitals Bristol NHS Foundation Trust.
Reproduced with permission.

CHAPTER 10

Activity 10.1

1 Nasal cavity
2 Pharynx
3 Epiglottis
4 Larynx
5 Trachea
6 Carina
7 Right main bronchus
8 Left Main bronchus
9 Alveoli (air sacs)
10 Diaphragm

Chapter 10 Test Your Knowledge

This student has opted to answer the question firstly by giving some background information on latex allergy as a whole, before describing the types of reactions. There has also been an attempt to compare and contrast the different allergy types. Some of the contents warranted an explanation, i.e. what is a T-cell-mediated and B-cell-mediated IgE response? Also, why are patients with spina bifida or having undergone urological or multiple surgery particularly susceptible to Type I allergy? The second part of the answer brought in directly the relevance in health care of latex allergy. All in all, it is quite a good answer. The word count was in the acceptable range of ±10% of 500 words. How did yours compare?

In order to answer the question, it is deemed necessary to firstly define the term 'latex allergy'. It is specifically an allergen in natural rubber latex from the *Heavea brasiliensis* tree that causes natural rubber latex allergy. A latex allergy is an immune response to latex and has been found to affect 15% of health workers in the USA. UK figures are unknown but estimates suggest 1% of the population. Those working in healthcare (and the hairdressing industry) are particularly at risk due to increased exposure to latex and nitrile (non-latex) gloves.

There are two types of latex allergy; Type IV hypersensitivity and a Type I hypersensitivity.

Type IV allergy is due to a sensitisation to the chemicals used in manufacturing causing contact dermatitis or a chemical allergy. There is a delayed reaction post-exposure of 6–48 hours due to T-cell mediated immune response causing a localised response causing skin dryness and blisters due to contact dermatitis. Type IV allergy is not life-threatening.

Type I allergy is due to B-cell mediated 1gE immune response. This type of allergy is more immediate (5–30 minutes) and can be life-threatening. Individuals with spina bifida, urological or multiple surgery are particularly susceptible.

Signs and symptoms of Type I Allergy are:

- Urticaria
- Itchy eyes
- Swelling of the lips and tongue
- Breathlessness
- Abdominal pain
- Hypotension
- Anaphylaxis
- In worse cases – death

(continued)

Individuals with a Type I allergy will need to be closely observed for 'Latex fruit syndrome' as the protein causing the allergy are similar to proteins found in certain fruits (known as 'cross-reactive allergens'). These fruits are avocadoes, apples, bananas, celery, cherries, chestnuts, ficus, figs, grapes, kiwi fruit, mangoes, melons, passion fruit, peaches, pears, pistachios, ragweed, strawberries and tomatoes.

For Type I and Type IV allergies, staff working in a healthcare environment should be reported to occupation health and should avoid exposure to the material causing problems (latex or chemicals used in manufacturing).

Other management strategies for Type I allergy should include the individual wearing a Medi-alert bracelet or necklace and carrying an Epipen containing adrenaline. These individuals should avoid the cross-reactive allergens, as above.

In healthcare, it is the responsibility of staff to protect those with an allergy, be these patients or staff members. Patients should be educated in latex allergy.

Within the healthcare environment, there are many latex products, such as blood-pressure cuffs, rubber bungs on drug ampoules, rubber ports on IV administration sets and syringes. Each ward, department, theatre, nursing home and GP's surgery should stock latex-free alternative products with staff being informed of the location of this equipment. Also, gloves should only be worn when necessary and hands should be washed flowing glove removal.

Communication and education is key in avoiding our patients being exposed to latex and this should be communicated to all staff members and documented in all notes and care plans.

To conclude, there are two types of natural rubber latex allergy – Type I (due to latex proteins) and Type IV (due to chemicals) and health carers have a duty of care to protect individuals from exposure to latex allergens and cross-reactive allergens found in medical equipment and fruits.

Word count: 529

CHAPTER 11
Activity 11.1
This reflection will be personal to you.

Chapter 11 Test Your Knowledge
The SWOT analysis and piece of reflection will be personal to you.

CHAPTER 12
Activity 12.1
1   Observation of patient contact
2   Observation of communication skills
3   Role-model observation
4   Observation of team-working

5   Context based learning
6   Experience of real clinical medical conditions, preparing the student for the sort of work they may encounter at a later date once qualified

CHAPTER 13
Chapter 13 Test Your Knowledge
1   Social health, physical health, psychological health
2   The holistic approach to health
3   Communing with nature; thought to decrease stress
4   Now, look at your next assignment and start planning!

APPENDICES

Appendix 1

Examples of Question Frameworks

PICOT   PICO + **T** (timeframe)

PICOC   PICO + **C** (context)

PICOTT   PICO + **TT** (TT refers to the *type* of question and the best *type* of study design)

PESICO   **P**opulation, **E**nvironment, **S**takeholders, **I**ntervention, **C**omparison, **O**utcome

PIPOH   **P**opulation, **I**ntervention, **P**rofessionals, **O**utcome, **H**ealthcare setting

ECLIPSE   **E**xpectation, **Cl**ient group, **L**ocation, **I**mpact, **P**rofessionals, **Se**rvice (addresses questions related to health policy and management)

Appendix 2
Glossary of Evidence Types

case-control study

A study which involves identifying patients who have the outcome of interest (cases) and control patients without the same outcome, and looking back to see if they had the exposure of interest.

case series

A report on a series of patients with an outcome of interest. No control group is involved.

cohort study

Involves identification of two groups (cohorts) of patients (e.g. people with asthma), one that received the 'exposure of interest' (such as being exposed to indoor smoking), and one that did not, and following these cohorts forward for the outcome of interest.

meta-analysis

A systematic review that uses quantitative methods to synthesize and summarise results.

randomized controlled trial (RCT)

Participants are randomly allocated into an experimental group or a control group and followed over time for the variables/outcomes of interest.

systematic review

A summary of the clinical literature that uses explicit methods to perform a comprehensive literature search and critical appraisal of individual studies and that may use appropriate statistical techniques to combine these valid studies when appropriate. The statistical technique for pooling studies is called a **meta-analysis**.

Source: Strauss, S.E., Glasziou, P., Richardson, W.S. and Haynes, R.B. (2011) *Evidence-Based Medicine: How to Practice and Teach It*, 4th edn. Churchill Livingstone, London; Appendix: Glossary pp. 269–273.

Appendix 3
Help with Analysis of Results

There are four parts to appraising statistics in papers and reports, as follows.

1   Is the analysis correct? (Usually impossible to determine without the full data set.)
2   Do I understand the statistical methods/analysis?
3   Do I understand the reporting of the results?
4   Are the conclusions appropriate given the strength and significance of the findings?

Statistical caveats

1   Probability is not proof.
2   Statistical significance is not the same as clinical significance.
3   Is the sample size sufficient to support the statistics? Think real people rather than numbers!
4   Do the statistics support the conclusions that the researchers have drawn?
5   Can you trust the statistics?

Books

Peat, J.K., Barton, B. and Elliott, E.J. (2008) *Statistics Workbook for Evidence-Based Health Care.* Wiley-Blackwell, Oxford.
Walker, J. and Almond, P. (2010) *Interpreting Statistical Findings: a Guide for Health Professionals and Students.* Open University Press, Maidenhead.

Final help with analysing data: ask a statistician!

Appendix 4

The New NHS in 2013: What it Means for You

The changes in the NHS aim to empower patients and local clinicians to make decisions about NHS services in your area.

Patients in England now have more choice and control over where to go for treatment, and can use patient power to make services better.

This infographic explains how the new NHS is structured.

Source: reproduced with permission of NHS Employers. © NHS Employers 2013.

Using the NHS

Monitori

Department of Health (DH)
The DH supports the Secretary of State for Health, setting national policy and legislation.

NHS England
NHS England is an independent body managing the NHS budget and commissioning services.

Clinical commissioning groups (CCGs)
Most of the NHS commissioning budget is now managed by 211 CCGs.

NHS Trust Development Authority (NHS TDA)
The NHS TDA provides governance and accountability for NHS trusts in England, and helps trusts prepare for foundation trust status.

Health and wellbeing boards
These are forums where key leaders from the health and care system work together to improve the health and wellbeing of their local population and reduce health inequalities.

Your local NHS
58 mental health trusts, providing services for people with mental health problems

36 community trusts, providing district nurses, health visitors for new parents and end-of-life care

11 ambulance trusts, operating the ambulance service across England, and making over 50,000 emergency journeys each week

2,312 hospitals (in the UK)
10,500 GP practices (in the UK)
10,000 dental practices (in the UK)
12,000 registered optometrists (in the UK)
10,000 pharmacies, providing a range of advisory services and dispensing of prescriptions.

Care Quality Commission (CQC)
The CQC is the independent regul of all health and social care service in England. Its job is to make sur that care provided meets nationa standards of quality and safety.

Healthwatch Englan
Healthwatch England is the independent consumer champion for health and social care in Engl Working with a network of 152

FACTS

Both men and women live an average of **ten years longer** than they did before the creation of the NHS.

Approximately 170,000 people (the capacity of the Glastonbury music festival) go for an eyesight test each week.

In 2010, 926.7 million prescriptions were dispensed and £3.8 billion was spent by the NHS on medicines used in hospitals.

The NHS deals with over 1 million patients every 36 hours.

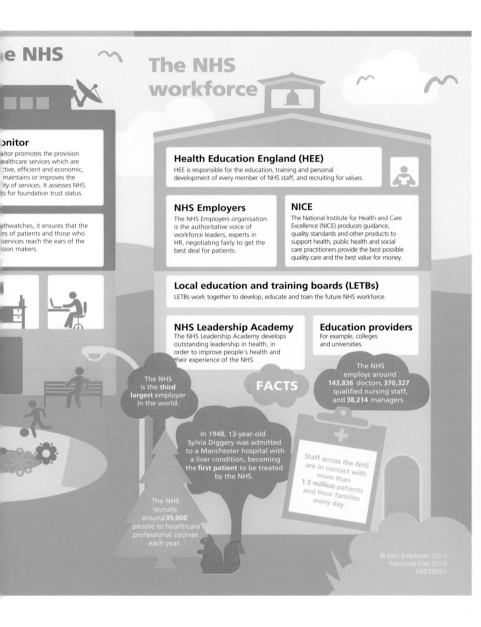

e NHS

onitor

itor promotes the provision
ealthcare services which are
ctive, efficient and economic,
maintains or improves the
ity of services. It assesses NHS
ts for foundation trust status.

thwatches, it ensures that the
es of patients and those who
services reach the ears of the
sion makers.

The NHS workforce

Health Education England (HEE)
HEE is responsible for the education, training and personal
development of every member of NHS staff, and recruiting for values.

NHS Employers
The NHS Employers organisation
is the authoritative voice of
workforce leaders, experts in
HR, negotiating fairly to get the
best deal for patients.

NICE
The National Institute for Health and Care
Excellence (NICE) produces guidance,
quality standards and other products to
support health, public health and social
care practitioners provide the best possible
quality care and the best value for money.

Local education and training boards (LETBs)
LETBs work together to develop, educate and train the future NHS workforce.

NHS Leadership Academy
The NHS Leadership Academy develops
outstanding leadership in health, in
order to improve people's health and
their experience of the NHS.

Education providers
For example, colleges
and universities.

The NHS
employs around
143,836 doctors, **370,327**
qualified nursing staff,
and **38,214** managers.

The NHS
is the **third
largest** employer
in the world.

FACTS

In 1948, 13-year-old
Sylvia Diggery was admitted
to a Manchester hospital with
a liver condition, becoming
the **first patient** to be treated
by the NHS.

Staff across the NHS
are in contact with
more than
1.5 million patients
and their families
every day.

The NHS
recruits
around **35,000**
people to healthcare
professional courses
each year.

© NHS Employers 2013
Published May 2013
EINF28501

Index

Study Skills for Nurses, First Edition. Claire Boyd and contributing author, Beverley Murray.
© 2014 John Wiley & Sons, Ltd. Published 2014 by John Wiley & Sons Ltd.

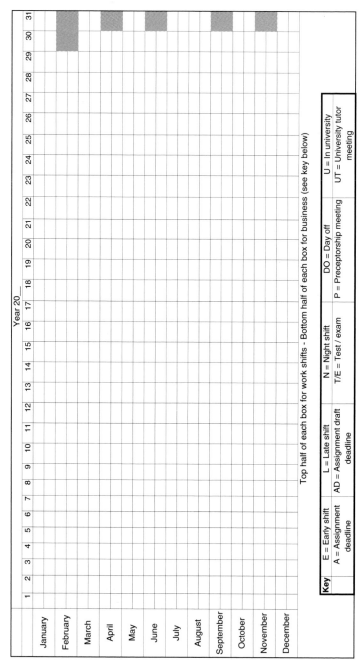

Year 20___

	1	2	3	4	5	6	7	8	9	10	11	12	13	14	15	16	17	18	19	20	21	22	23	24	25	26	27	28	29	30	31
January																															
February																															
March																															
April																															
May																															
June																															
July																															
August																															
September																															
October																															
November																															
December																															

Top half of each box for work shifts - Bottom half of each box for business (see key below)

Key	E = Early shift	L = Late shift	N = Night shift	DO = Day off	U = In university
	A = Assignment deadline	AD = Assignment draft deadline	T/E = Test / exam	P = Preceptorship meeting	UT = University tutor meeting

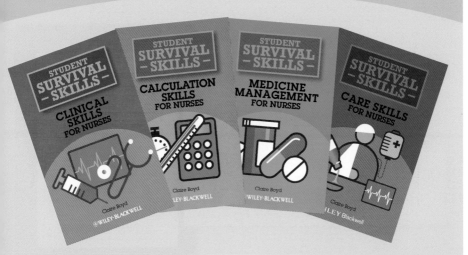
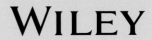

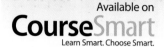
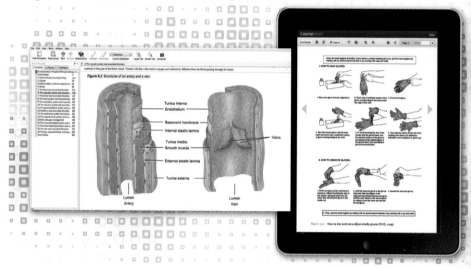